DIABETIC
RETINOPATHY

FROM DIAGNOSIS TO TREATMENT

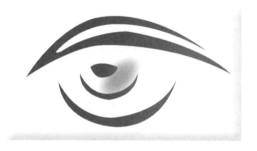

Homayoun Tabandeh, M.D.
David S. Boyer, M.D.

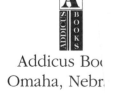

Addicus Bo[
Omaha, Nebr[

3\14
Brr

An Addicus Nonfiction Book

ISBN 978-1-936374-44-1

This book is not intended to be a substitute for a physician, nor do the authors intend to give advice contrary to that of an attending physician.

Noted photos within the book are courtesy of Thieme Publications. Homayoun Tabandeh, M.D., Morton F. Goldberg, M.D. *The Retina in Systemic Disease: A Color Manual of Opthalmoscopy,* 2009, Copyright by Homayoun Tabandeh, M.D., and Morton F. Goldberg, M.D., www.thieme.com. (*Reprinted with permission.*)

Library of Congress Cataloging-in-Publication Data

Boyer, David S., 1947
 Diabetic retinopathy : from diagnosis to treatment / David Boyer, Homayoun Tabandeh.
  p. cm.
 Includes bibliographical references and index.
 ISBN 978-1-936374-44-1 (alk. paper)
 1. Diabetic retinopathy. 2. Diabetic retinopathy—Treatment.
 I. Tabandeh, Homayoun. II. Title.
 RE661.D5B69 2013
 617.7'35--dc23
                                        2012031455

Addicus Books, Inc.
P.O. Box 45327
Omaha, Nebraska 68145
www.AddicusBooks.com

Printed in the United States of America
10 9 8 7 6 5 4 3 2 1

To the many people who are affected by diabetic retinopathy; to our patients, who entrusted their care to us and inspired us to write this book; to many colleagues who graciously entrusted us with their patient's care; and to our families, whose support made this project possible.

Contents

Acknowledgments

We are grateful to our patients, who, through sharing their experiences, have educated us to recognize the challenges they face daily. We hope this book will help those with diabetic retinopathy better understand their condition and make better-informed decisions through educating themselves on this important disease.

We would like to express our gratitude to the many colleagues who graciously entrusted us with their patients' care. We would like to thank Adam Smucker, Dr. Michelle Carle, and all the employees at the L.A. Retina-Vitreous Associates Medical Group, whose hard work and dedication to patient care have helped our patients and us tremendously. Our thanks also go to Christine Hinz and Rod Colvin at Addicus Books for their expert support of this project.

Introduction

Diabetes can affect the eye in many different ways. The most serious and common eye complication of diabetes is diabetic retinopathy. Diabetic retinopathy is the leading cause of vision loss in the working-age population. The American Diabetes Association estimates that 12,000 to 24,000 individuals with diabetes lose their eyesight each year due to the disease. Caused by changes in the blood vessels of the retina, diabetic retinopathy is a potential problem for people with either type 1 or type 2 diabetes. Without proper diagnosis and treatment it can do irreversible damage to your eyesight, sometimes before you even notice.

As retina specialists, we diagnose and treat patients with diabetic retinopathy every day. The number of individuals suffering vision problems associated with this eye condition is rising, not surprising given the epidemic increase in diabetes, its underlying cause.

If you or someone you know has been diagnosed with diabetic retinopathy, you will likely have many questions, both about the disease and the hurdles that may be encountered in the future. This book is a comprehensive, yet concise and easy-to-read, overview of both *nonproliferative* and *proliferative diabetic retinopathy,* the two major forms of this disease. We explore the causes, symptoms, and current treatments. Although no cure exists for diabetic retinopathy, today's therapies offer hope to millions of patients. Your eye specialist cannot reverse the damage that has already occurred, but he or she can help preserve your remaining vision.

It is our hope that this book will help you understand diabetic retinopathy and reduce the risk of damage to your vision.

Diabetic Retinopathy: An Overview

1

If you have type 1 or type 2 diabetes, you are at risk for developing diabetic retinopathy. According to the National Eye Institute, between 40 and 45 percent of Americans with diabetes have some form of *diabetic retinopathy,* the most common eye condition linked to diabetes.

In the United States, the Centers for Disease Control and Prevention reports between 12,000 and 24,000 new cases of blindness each year due to diabetic retinopathy, making it the leading cause of vision loss among American adults between the ages of twenty and seventy-four. The Center also projects that by 2050, the number of Americans ages forty and older affected by diabetic retinopathy will grow from a current 5 million individuals to about 16 million. Although these statistics are alarming, you can prevent or delay damage to your vision by controlling your diabetes along with getting regular eye evaluations and treatment.

Defining *Diabetic Retinopathy*

Diabetic retinopathy is a disease of the retina caused by diabetes. It usually affects both eyes and occurs when uncontrolled blood sugar levels damage

1

Eye Anatomy

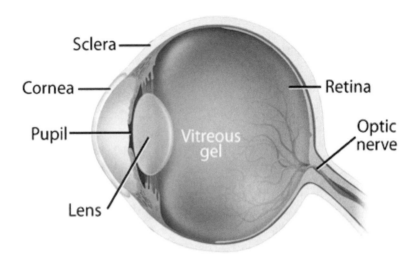

the small vessels of the *retina,* the light-sensitive tissue in the back of your eye. The retina is responsible for processing images that make vision possible. To produce clear, distortion-free vision, the retina must receive an abundant supply of oxygen and nutrients. If the blood vessels to the retina are damaged as a result of diabetes, the retina becomes deprived of essential nutrients and will not function correctly. The delicate retina tissue is gradually damaged, and images that you see may be blurred or otherwise distorted.

Diabetic retinopathy is a progressive disease—it worsens over time. Although some effects, such as blurriness and distortion, may be mild or short-term, other complications can cause severe, long-term vision loss.

Symptoms of Diabetic Retinopathy

Because diabetic retinopathy rarely causes pain, symptoms are not always apparent in the early stages. In fact, damage to your retina could be occurring long before you have noticeable signs. When symptoms do occur, they are often caused by retinopathy affecting the macula, the area of the retina responsible for central vision. Symptoms may include the following:

- blurred vision
- seeing dark spots or "floaters" (small specs in your field of vision)
- vision loss
- blind spots in your vision

It is important that you see your eye specialist as soon as possible if you have any such symptoms. Diabetic retinopathy cannot be cured, but with careful monitoring it can be diagnosed, treated, and controlled before it impairs your vision further.

Types of Diabetic Retinopathy

The main forms of diabetic retinopathy include nonproliferative diabetic retinopathy (NPDR), proliferative diabetic retinopathy (PDR), diabetic macular edema, and advanced diabetic eye disease.

Nonproliferative Diabetic Retinopathy

Nonproliferative diabetic retinopathy is an early form of the disease in which symptoms might be nonexistent or mild. Damage results from injury to the *capillaries,* small blood vessels of your retina. With nonproliferative diabetic retinopathy, damage to the retina may occur in two ways. First, the tiny

3

Nonproliferative Diabetic Retinopathy

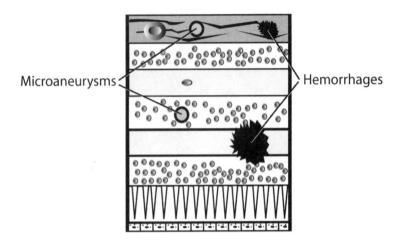

Microaneurysms — Hemorrhages

This illustration represents retina tissue. Nonproliferative diabetic retinopathy occurs when tiny blood vessels in the retina are damaged as a result of poor blood sugar control. The dark patches represent tiny hemorrhages.

vessels weaken, and eventually leak blood and fluid into the retina. Second, blockage of small blood-vessel networks may result in areas of the retina becoming deprived of oxygen and nutrients. This leads to a cycle of more retinal tissue damage and more abnormal leakage from the blood vessels.

Eye specialists classify nonproliferative diabetic retinopathy as mild, moderate, or severe depending on the amount of retinal abnormalities they see during a retina examination. These stages of the disease are described in the text that follows.

Mild nonproliferative diabetic retinopathy. This phase occurs when retinal blood vessels first weaken and leak. Tiny bulges, known as *microaneurysms,* protrude from the vessel walls. At the same time,

The Human Eyeball: Similar to a Camera

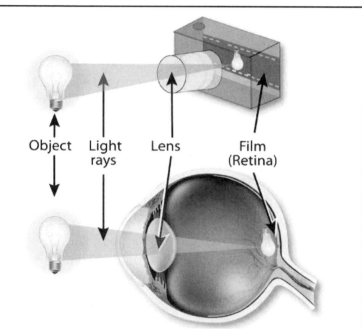

Object — Light rays — Lens — Film (Retina)

The eyeball lens is a focusing system, similar to a camera lens. The retina, tissue lining the back of the eye, functions as the camera's "film." The retina carries signals (images we see) along the optic nerve to the brain, where they are interpreted as vision.

The macula, the area at the center of the retina, allows you to see fine details and recognize colors. A dimple, known as the fovea, at the center of the macula makes sharp vision possible.

The peripheral retina, which is the portion of the retina that is outside the macula, is responsible for your side vision. It also makes night vision possible. The space between the retina and the lens, the vitreous, is filled with clear gel that enables the eyeball to hold its shape.

The retina receives oxygen and nutrients through two different networks of blood vessels—the retinal blood vessels and choroid blood vessels. The choroid is a carpet of blood vessels that nourishes the outside layer of the retina.

retinal hemorrhages, tiny "dots" or "blotches," leak from the capillaries into the retina while protein and lipid deposits, called *hard exudates,* form on the retina. They look like tiny waxy white or yellow flecks. Although an ophthalmologist can see these flecks during an eye examination, you may not notice any symptoms at this point, unless the center of your macula is involved.

Moderate nonproliferative diabetic retinopathy. This stage of retinopathy occurs as more hemorrhages and microaneurysms form. Small vessels that normally nourish the retina actually may become blocked or closed. These obstructions may cause a decrease in the supply of oxygen and nutrient-rich blood to the retina, particularly to the macula, in what is called *retinal* or *macular ischemia.* The oxygen loss prevents the macula from working correctly and causes vision problems.

Severe nonproliferative diabetic retinopathy. This stage is characterized by more extensive retinal hemorrhages, microaneurysms, dilation of blood vessels, and opening of blood vessels called "intraretinal microvascular abnormalities." Because many more retinal blood vessels are blocked or closed during this stage of nonproliferative diabetic retinopathy, larger areas of the retina are deprived of necessary oxygen and nutrients. In an attempt to reestablish the oxygen supply and nourishment, the retina produces special chemicals that trigger growth of new blood vessels. Increased production of these chemicals also causes the retinal blood vessels to leak more and build up fluid in the retina, particularly in the macula.

Proliferative Diabetic Retinopathy

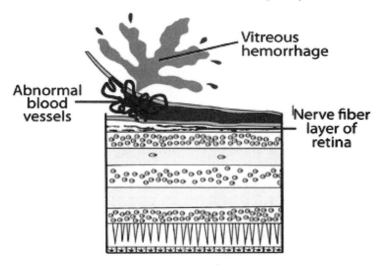

With proliferative diabetic retinopathy, abnormal blood vessels may grow and bleed into the vitreous gel. This is known as a vitreous hemorrhage.

Proliferative Diabetic Retinopathy (PDR)

A more advanced form of the disease, proliferative diabetic retinopathy occurs when the retina is so deprived of oxygenated blood that abnormal blood vessels grow or *proliferate* to accommodate the loss (this is called *retinal neovascularization*). It would seem that this *proliferation* would be nature's healing response; however, the new vessels are so fragile that they may break and bleed, causing scarring that may lead to loss of vision. Proliferative diabetic retinopathy carries with it the same problems associated with nonproliferative diabetic retinopathy, such as diabetic macular edema, along with several others, including diabetic macular edema, vitreous hemorrhage, retinal detachment, and neovascular glaucoma.

Diabetic Macular Edema

Diabetic macular edema refers to swelling of the macula (central part of the retina) caused by a buildup of leakage from blood vessels. Macular edema leads to blurring and loss of central vision, and it is the most common cause of blindness among those with diabetic retinopathy. Macular edema may occur with proliferative diabetic retinopathy or with nonproliferative diabetic retinopathy.

Diabetic Macular Edema

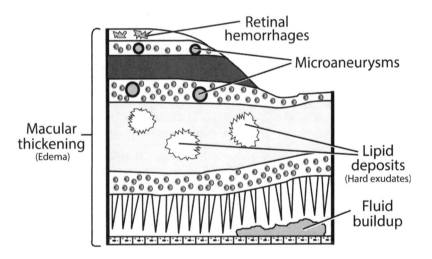

Excessive leakage from the retinal blood vessels causes the macula tissue to swell and thicken. Macular edema is the most common cause of vision loss with diabetic retinopathy.

Advanced Diabetic Eye Diseases

Vitreous Hemorrhage

A common complication of severe proliferative diabetic retinopathy, a *vitreous hemorrhage* refers to bleeding into the vitreous. As mentioned earlier, the vitreous is the clear gel that fills the space in the middle of the eye. It is situated between the lens in the front of the eye and the retina lining the back of the eye. There are normally no blood vessels within the vitreous gel.

Under normal circumstances, light rays pass through the vitreous to reach the retina. In proliferative diabetic retinopathy, however, fragile new vessels of the retina can rupture, clouding the once transparent vitreous gel with blood so those light rays cannot reach the retina. Although vitreous bleeding can cause vision problems, it usually does not trigger permanent vision loss. In many cases, proper treatment will restore vision.

Tractional Retinal Detachment

One of the most serious complications of proliferative diabetic retinopathy is a tractional retinal detachment. It occurs when scar tissue forms alongside new vessels. As the scarring shrinks and contracts, it pulls on the retina and its blood vessels. This contracting not only causes the vessels to bleed but also causes the retina to wrinkle. It may pull away from its normal position, tear, or completely detach. The wrinkling may distort your vision. If the macula or large retinal areas detach, you will likely experience greater vision loss. As a serious complication, trac-

9

Tractional Retinal Detachment

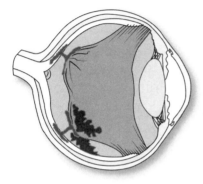

Prior to detachment, the tiny blood vessels leak into the vitreous gel.

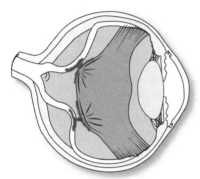

As the bleeding continues into the vitreous gel, it contracts and pulls on the retina, causing it to detach.

tional retinal detachment may require surgical correction to avoid progressive and permanent loss of vision.

Neovascular Glaucoma

Proliferative diabetic retinopathy is a risk factor for a severe type of glaucoma called *neovascular glaucoma*. This condition develops when new vessels growing over the iris block the normal flow of fluids away from the eye; this blockage causes severely elevated eye pressure. When the pressure inside the eye rises to higher levels, the optic nerve—which transfers visual information to the brain—is severely damaged. Symptoms of neovascular glaucoma include eye pain, redness, and loss of vision.

Risk Factors for Diabetic Retinopathy

There are many factors that can raise your risk for diabetic retinopathy. You will note, however, that many of these risk factors can be controlled.

Duration of Diabetes

The longer you have had poorly controlled blood glucose levels, the higher your risk for diabetic retinopathy. Most diabetic individuals develop eye problems over time, making duration of their diabetes one of the strongest predictors that they will develop this eye disease. Research has shown that nearly all type 1 diabetics and 60 percent of type 2 diabetics develop diabetic eye disease within the first two decades of their diabetes diagnosis.

The findings of the *Wisconsin Epidemiological Study of Diabetic Retinopathy,* which tracked complications in nearly 2,400 type 1 and type 2 diabetic individuals, supports the idea that the longer you have diabetes, the greater your chances for developing diabetic retinopathy. In the study, among younger-onset (type 1) diabetes patients alone, the prevalence of retinopathy was 8 percent at three years, 25 percent at five years, 60 percent at ten years, and 80 percent at fifteen years. By fifteen years, 25 percent of participants had advanced diabetic retinopathy.

According to the same study, up to 21 percent of type 2 diabetics have retinopathy when they're diagnosed with diabetes. Most patients develop some degree of it over time.

Summary of Stages of Diabetic Retinopathy
Mild Nonproliferative Retinopathy
At this earliest stage, microaneurysms occur. They are small areas of balloon-like swelling in the retina's tiny blood vessels.
Moderate Nonproliferative Retinopathy
As the disease progresses, some blood vessels that nourish the retina are blocked.
Severe Nonproliferative Retinopathy
Many more blood vessels are blocked, depriving several areas of the retina of their blood supply. These areas of the retina send signals to the body to grow new blood vessels for nourishment.
Proliferative Retinopathy
At this advanced stage, the signals sent by the retina for nourishment trigger the growth of new blood vessels. These new blood vessels are abnormal and fragile. They grow along the retina and along the surface of the clear, vitreous gel that fills the inside of the eye. By themselves, these blood vessels do not cause symptoms or vision loss. However, they have thin, fragile walls. If they leak blood, severe vision loss and even blindness can result.
Source: National Eye Institute, U.S. National Institutes of Health. www.nei.nih.gov

Poor Blood Glucose Control

In addition to the duration of your diabetes, controlling your blood glucose has a major bearing on your risk for diabetic retinopathy. Chronically high blood glucose levels, or *hyperglycemia,* damages your retinal vessels. The American Diabetes Association (ADA) recommends fasting glucose levels between 70 and 120 mg/dL and less than 180 mg/dL two hours after meals. The association also recommends a *hemoglobin A1c* (HA1c) of 7 percent or less. The hemoglobin A1c is a protein in red blood cells that bonds with blood sugars. Becasue red blood cells can live from 90 to 120 days, the hemoglobin A1c stays in the

Defining Diabetes

Diabetes mellitus, or simply diabetes, is a group of metabolic diseases in which the body does not metabolize glucose properly, resulting in high blood sugar. Glucose is the most commonly found type of sugar in the body. Under normal circumstances a number of hormones help regulate the glucose metabolism, the most important being insulin.

Insulin helps body cells take up and process sugar in to energy. Insulin is produced by the pancreas, a small gland sandwiched between the spine and stomach. In diabetes, there is either a deficiency of insulin production or an increased resistance to its effects, resulting in high levels of blood glucose. The chronically elevated blood glucose damages various organs of the body including the eye, the kidney, the nerves, and the blood vessels throughout the body. There are many types of diabetes, the main ones are type 1 diabetes and type 2 diabetes.

Type 1 diabetes occurs when the pancreas does not produce enough insulin. It usually develops during childhood or adolescence; it can also occur in adults, however. About 10 percent of those with diabetes have type 1. This form was previously referred to as insulin-dependent diabetes mellitus or juvenile diabetes. Those with type 1 diabetes need to take insulin injections or receive infusions from an insulin pump, which is worn; the pump may be attached to a waistband, pocket, bra, garter belt, sock, or underwear. Once produced from cow and pig pancreases, today's insulin is made from genetically engineered bacteria and manufactured in a laboratory.

Type 2 diabetes is the most common type of diabetes, affecting about 90 percent of those with diabetes. It results from insulin resistance, a condition in which cells fail to use insulin efficiently. As a result, blood glucose levels rise. This form of the disease is often referred to as adult-onset diabetes. Many individuals take oral medication; others may require daily insulin injections.

blood for that length of time. Accordingly, the HA1c provides a measurement of blood sugar control over the previous few months. This test tells doctors how well your treatment plan is working.

Obesity

The more fatty tissue you have, the more resistant your cells are to insulin. Obesity increases your risk for diabetes as well as other serious conditions such as high cholesterol and high blood pressure. Estimates suggest that 65 percent of Americans are overweight, meaning they have a body mass index (BMI) of 25 to 29. Body mass index is a measurement of one's percentage of body fat—the ratio between one's weight and one's height.

Using BMI does have its drawbacks. The formula doesn't consider lean body mass, so a muscular, heavy person may have a high BMI but be in terrific shape. For the vast majority of the population, however, BMI remains the best overall indicator of obesity.

Lifestyle Choices

A sedentary lifestyle, especially if you are overweight, contributes to many diseases, including diabetes, heart disease, high blood pressure, and high cholesterol levels. On the other hand, physical exercise improves circulation, lowers blood sugars, and improves your body's use of insulin. This results in improved blood sugar levels. This benefit of increased sensitivity to insulin continues for hours after you stop exercising.

Classification of Weight by BMI

BMI	Classification
less than 18.5	Underweight
18.5–24.9	Normal
25–29.9	Overweight
30–34.9	Class I Obesity
35–39.9	Class II Obesity
greater than 40	Class III Obesity
greater than 60	Super-Obesity

Exercise also promotes weight loss. A sedentary lifestyle contributes to insulin resistance, making it more difficult to keep weight off. Even light or moderate physical activity can help lower blood sugars.

Smoking is another major risk factor for developing diabetic retinopathy. Smoking also causes diabetic retinopathy to progress faster. The nicotine in tobacco not only contributes to higher blood pressure and higher cholesterol levels, but it also impairs insulin activity. Even though quitting smoking can be difficult, it is critical to heart health and diabetes control.

Unlike smoking, alcohol consumption doesn't have a direct influence on diabetic retinopathy. Yet, because it can affect diabetes control, drinking in excess can affect the health of your eyes. Your doctor can tell you what constitutes drinking in moderation.

High Cholesterol Levels
Diabetes puts you at risk for chronically high cholesterol or blood fats that promote the buildup of plaque in your arteries. Although the small vessels

of the retina are too small for such buildup, uncontrolled cholesterol can contribute to macular edema and the development of hard exudates, the small yellow spots or lipid deposits that may form in the retina. Both conditions are associated with a higher risk of vision loss.

Doctors advise keeping "bad" or low-density cholesterol (LDLs) less than 70 mg/dL. "Good" cholesterol or high-density lipoproteins (HDLs) should be greater than 40 mg/dL in men and 50 mg/dL in women. Both men and women should strive for triglycerides, another type of fat, at levels less than 150 mg/dL.

High Blood Pressure

If you have both diabetes and high blood pressure (also called *hypertension*), you are at higher risk for a number of eye-related problems, including retinopathy, glaucoma, and optic nerve damage. Elevated blood pressure not only stresses your heart, it also raises the chance for eye problems, particularly macular edema and bleeding. Chronic hypertension combined with long-term diabetes also increases the chance that your retinopathy will be more destructive and progress more quickly. Research consistently shows that keeping your blood pressure below 130/80 mmHg protects your eyes as well as your heart.

Race/Ethnicity

Diabetic retinopathy is more common in some ethnic and racial groups than in others. African Americans, Asian Americans, Hispanic/Latino Americans,

American Indians, and Alaskan Natives are at higher risk for type 2 diabetes than non-Hispanic whites. African Americans and Hispanic individuals are almost twice as likely as whites to have eye problems, according to the American Diabetes Association. Researchers are not sure why some ethnic groups have higher rates of diabetes, which increase the risk for retinopathy and other problems.

Age and Gender

As mentioned earlier, the longer you have diabetes, the greater your risk for diabetic retinopathy. Not surprisingly, this complication is rare among children but common among older diabetic adults. A recent study by *Prevent Blindness America* and the National Eye Institute demonstrated that older adult Americans are facing a bigger threat of all age-related eye diseases (diabetic retinopathy, age-related macular degeneration, cataracts, and open-angle glaucoma) today than at any other time.

Genetics

Genetics determine many things about us, including our predisposition for certain health issues such as diabetes. A family history of type 2 diabetes significantly increases the risk of an individual developing type 2 diabetes. Scientists believe that individual genes or combinations of them either promote diabetes in certain individuals or protect them from developing it. Scientists have yet to identify every gene involved in type 1 and type 2 diabetes, but they know that genetics are a factor. Research studies of identical twins, for instance, have demonstrated that if one twin has type 1 diabetes, the other twin has a 50 percent change of developing the disease. If one twin has type 2 diabetes, the other twin has a 75 percent chance of developing it.

Pregnancy

Gestational diabetes is a type of diabetes linked to pregnancy; diabetic retinopathy is usually not a complication in these women. If, however, you already have diabetic retinopathy and become pregnant, you are at risk: diabetic retinopathy can progress rapidly during pregnancy because the hormonal and metabolic changes of pregnancy can make the disease and its complications worse. It is recommended that you see a retina specialist if you have diabetic retinopathy and become pregnant. You may need monitoring throughout the pregnancy.

Other Eye Conditions Affected by Diabetes

If you have diabetes, you are at risk for eye problems beyond diabetic retinopathy. For instance, if your sugar levels rise and fall, the fluctuations can cause the lens of the eye to swell, triggering blurriness and other distortions. Even though you may not have diabetic retinopathy, such lens problems can cause symptoms at any stage of disease. You may find your vision fluctuating during the course of the day.

Glaucoma

As mentioned earlier, glaucoma is a serious eye disease in which pressure inside the eye gradually builds up, causing damage to the optic nerve. This process occurs because natural fluid secreted by the eye cannot exit properly. Instead, it collects within the eyeball, triggering an increase in eye pressure that may affect vision.

According to the American Diabetes Association, if you have diabetes, you are more likely to develop glaucoma than individuals without diabetes. There are several types of glaucoma. The three major types are *open-angle glaucoma, closed-angle glaucoma,* and *neovascular glaucoma.*

Open-angle or *chronic glaucoma* is the most common form of the disease. With this form, the space or angle between the iris and the cornea does not drain fluid efficiently. Instead, fluid collects, causing pressure to rise and gradually damage the optic nerve. This may lead to a slow loss of peripheral vision, your side vision, that ultimately may result in tunnel vision. Open-angle glaucoma is also called chronic because it happens over time.

Acute closed-angle glaucoma is the less common form of the disease. Here, the fluid drainage space itself is blocked, usually because the bulging iris narrows the space. Yet, the eye continues to secrete fluid. But because the fluid is trapped, it causes a sudden increase in pressure, which can lead to optic nerve damage. The symptoms include severe eye pain and loss of vision.

A less common but equally serious form of glaucoma is *neovascular glaucoma*. As explained previously, neovascular glaucoma results when abnormal new blood vessels grow over the iris and into the drainage space; this blocks the drainage of the fluid from inside of the eye. As the fluid collects, pressure builds, eventually damaging the optic nerve.

Symptoms of neovascular glaucoma come on quickly and include:

- severe eye pain
- eye redness
- headache
- nausea and vomiting
- loss of vision

If you experience these or other symptoms that may indicate neovascular glaucoma or other forms of glaucoma, see your eye specialist immediately. Time is of the essence for saving your sight.

Cataracts

Cataracts, or clouding of the lens that can dim or distort vision, is a common occurrence in older Americans. But if you have diabetes, you are 60 percent more likely to develop a cataract than nondiabetic individuals, according to the American Diabetes Association. You are also more likely to develop a type of cataract called a *posterior subcapsular cataract,* which is often related to poor blood glucose control. Such cataracts develop in a critical position at the back of the lens and block the path of light traveling to the retina. Because of this location, posterior subcapsular cataracts can be small yet still cause significant visual problems.

Diabetes-related cataracts can occur as early as age thirty or forty. They also progress more rapidly than the cataracts associated with normal aging. You may not have symptoms at the very earliest stage of any cataract. As the cloudiness develops, however, you will likely experience:

- blurred, doubled, or dimmed vision
- sensitivity to bright lights or glare
- "halos" around lights
- fading or yellowing of colors
- frequent changes in your eyeglass or contact lens prescription

Your symptoms will make reading and other detailed work difficult. You also may have problems driving at night because oncoming lights produce a blinding glare.

Optic Neuropathy

The optic nerve contains more than 1 million nerve fibers; as mentioned earlier, this nerve is responsible for transmitting images to our brain, which in turn interprets what the object is. Diabetic retinopathy is a risk factor for *optic neuropathy*, a condition caused by an insufficient blood supply to the optic nerve. The lack of blood supply may be made worse by a drop in blood pressure. Optic neuropathy is like having a "stroke" in the optic nerve. Damage to the optic nerve may cause serious vision loss.

Retinal Vein Occlusion

A retinal vein occlusion is a blockage of the veins that carry blood away from the retina. It may cause painless loss of vision, retinal hemorrhages, and in severe cases macular edema and retinal neovacularization, which is the formation of tiny, fragile blood vessels in the retina.

Corneal Problems

The cornea is a thin, clear layer of tissue on the surface of the eye. Light rays pass through the cornea to the retina in the back of the eye. Recurrent corneal erosion is a problem seen more frequently in persons with diabetes. This typically causes episodes of severe sharp eye pain as the front layer of the cornea (corneal epithelium) becomes loose. The condition often subsides spontaneously before recurring at a later date. Treatment is required if the condition becomes severe or occurs frequently.

In Summary

- Educating yourself about diabetes and the problems associated with it is an effective first step in controlling this condition.
- Diabetic retinopathy is a serious complication of diabetes that results from high glucose levels damaging the retinal blood vessels. This can cause loss of vision.
- Between 40 and 45 percent of Americans with diabetes have some form of diabetic retinopathy.

- With time, diabetic retinopathy progresses to mild, moderate, and then severe nonproliferative diabetic retinopathy.

- Without proper diagnosis and treatment, nonproliferative diabetic retinopathy can advance to proliferative diabetic retinopathy, which is a serious sight-threatening stage of the disease.

- Macular edema is due to buildup of fluid, which results in thickening of the macula and can occur in any type of diabetic retinopathy, leading to loss of vision.

- The duration of your diabetes and how well your blood glucose is controlled are major risk factors for the development and progression of diabetic retinopathy.

- Other risk factors that play a significant role, also in common to heart disease, include obesity, high blood pressure, high cholesterol, and smoking. Risk factors that you cannot control include race/ethnicity, age, gender, and genetics.

- Individuals with diabetes are also at increased risk for other eye diseases, especially glaucoma, cataracts, retinal vein occlusion, optic nerve damage, and corneal problems.

- Good blood sugar control, regular eye examination, and timely treatment are the key factors in reducing damage to the eye and keeping your vision.

2 Getting a Diagnosis

Your eye care specialist will perform a variety of tests to determine whether you have diabetic retinopathy. These test results will determine the stage of your eye disease. Diabetic retinopathy is classified as mild, moderate, or severe nonproliferative diabetic retinopathy or proliferative diabetic retinopathy, which is the more serious type. Diabetic retinopathy can occur in both type 1 and type 2 diabetes.

During a comprehensive eye exam, the specialist will also be checking for other possible eye conditions such as cataracts and glaucoma. You may find it helpful to have a basic understanding of the types of eye care professionals you may see and types of diagnostic procedures you may undergo as part of your evaluation.

Eye Care Professionals

Selecting the right eye care professional is important. Several types of health professionals are skilled in diagnosing eye problems, including diabetic retinopathy. *Optometrists* and *general ophthalmologists* practice general eye care. They are often the first to notice diabetic retinopathy. If you are found to have retinal changes related to your diabetes, you'll likely be referred to a retina specialist, an expert in diagnosing and treating diseases of the retina and macula. Let's take a closer look at the role each of these professionals play in eye care.

Optometrists

Also referred to as *optometric doctors (O.D.)*, optometrists are trained to perform routine eye exams, prescribe eyeglasses or contact lenses, and diagnose ocular problems. To be licensed, an optometrist must have earned a college degree and then completed four years of training at an accredited optometry school. If your optometrist suspects diabetic retinopathy or a related eye problem, he or she may refer you to an ophthalmologist or retina specialist.

General Ophthalmologists

An ophthalmologist is a physician who has first earned a bachelor's degree and completed medical school before graduating with an M.D. or doctor of medicine degree. Ophthalmologists then complete one year of internship and three years of additional training (residency training) focused entirely on the eye. After they complete their residency training and have successfully completed an ophthalmology specialty examination, they are certified by the American Board of Ophthalmology. After obtaining state medical licensure, general ophthalmologists are qualified to perform eye surgery. If ophthalmologists see signs of diabetic retinopathy, they may refer you to a retina specialist for further testing and treatment.

Retina Specialists

Retina specialists are ophthalmologists with extensive training in diagnosing and treating retinal problems such as diabetic retinopathy and macular degeneration. They have received two years of additional education (called a *fellowship*) after becoming ophthalmologists. Retina specialists are skilled in using advanced imaging and other examination tools to evaluate the health of the retina. They perform laser procedures, *intravitreal injections,* and complex surgical procedures for a variety of conditions, including diabetic retinopathy.

Preparing for Your Examination

For your eye specialist to make an accurate diagnosis, he or she needs your help. You'll want to go to your consultation with details of your medical history, especially information pertaining to your diabetes and any previous eye problems. Your doctor will want to know about such things as:

- health conditions, past and present
- any past or present eye disorders, injuries, or surgeries
- prescription medications you currently take
- your use of over-the-counter medications, including vitamins, supplements, herbs, and homeopathic products
- any allergies to medication
- smoking history, past and present
- alcohol consumption, past and present

- family medical history, including general medical problems and eye conditions
- your primary care and diabetes doctors' contact information

After reviewing your general health, your eye specialist will proceed with examining your eyes. With diabetic retinopathy, you may or may not experience symptoms of the disease, especially in its earliest stages. It is important, however, to provide as much information to your eye care specialist as possible. It will be helpful to the specialist if you can supply information about:

- any changes in your vision or symptoms— such as "floaters," wavy lines, blurriness, or dark or empty spots in your central vision
- approximate time frame you first noticed the symptoms
- conditions under which you experience symptoms. Are they intermittent or constant? Do they occur under certain conditions, such as dimmed light?
- your symptom progression. Are symptoms getting worse?

Remember to take your contact lenses and any eyeglasses—both for distance and reading—to your appointment. It's also a good idea to take sunglasses because your eyes will be sensitive to bright light after they've been dilated for your examination. If possible, you should plan to ask someone to drive you to and from the appointment.

Your Eye Examination

A routine eye exam may be as brief as half an hour, but a comprehensive exam for the diagnosis of diabetic retinopathy may take two or more hours. The length of your exam depends on several factors, including which diagnostic tests are needed and any possible treatments that you may receive during the appointment. Following are some of the tests that may be part of your examination.

Visual Acuity Testing

Visual acuity refers to the clarity of your central vision, or simply put, how well you see. With all of the high-tech diagnostic tools available to eye doctors today, the tool most commonly used to test visual acuity is low-tech—it's the Snellen visual acuity chart, the basic eye chart developed in the nineteenth century. During a vision test, the chart is usually read from a distance of twenty feet. You have probably heard the expression, "20-20 vision"; the first number refers to reading the chart from twenty feet. The second number indicates how much your visual acuity differs from a normal healthy eye. For example, if you have 20/20 vision—which is considered ideal—you are able to identify objects or letters that a person with normal eyesight can identify from twenty feet away.

If your vision is 20/40, this indicates that what people with good vision can identify from forty feet away must be brought closer, to twenty feet in front of you, in order for you to be able to identify it. The higher the second number, the worse your visual acuity.

When checking your visual acuity, your eye care specialist will test each eye separately. It is not uncommon for one eye to have better vision than the other.

Testing Eye Pressure

Testing the pressure inside the eyes is commonly performed to screen for glaucoma, a condition that causes a build-up of pressure inside the eye; this pressure can damage the optic nerve. Glaucoma is not a sign of diabetic retinopathy; measuring eye pressure is, however, an important part of a comprehensive eye exam. Your eye care professional may use one of a number of methods to test eye pressure.

Goldmann tonometry. In this commonly used test, a nurse or technician puts a drop of yellow dye along with topical anesthetic in your eye. You are then asked to place your chin on the chin rest of a device called a *slit lamp*. A slit lamp is a modified microscope with a bright light that allows an eye care specialist to view the eye under high magnification. The head of a small pressure sensor is gently placed against the surface of your eye. Then, the pressure reading is done under blue light, which illuminates the dye.

Snellen Eye Chart

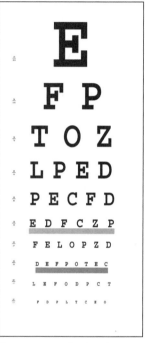

Eye care professionals use the Snellen eye chart to test visual acuity. It is usually read from a distance of twenty feet.

Tono-Pen. Nowadays, many doctors use a newer device to measure the eye pressure. It's called a Tono-Pen, which looks like a ballpoint pen. With this method, anesthetic eyedrops are used to numb the surface of your eye. The tip of the Tono-Pen is then gently placed against the eyeball and a digital readout displays the eye pressure measurement.

With both of these methods, the eyes are tested individually. If your eye pressure is high, you may be at risk for glaucoma.

Visual Field Testing

Visual field testing refers to checking areas of central and peripheral vision. As mentioned previously, peripheral vision is your "side vision"—your ability to see objects that are not in your direct line of vision. A visual field test is performed as you look at a small, central point while lights of various sizes are projected at various locations. You are asked to indicate each time you see the light.

Testing Range of Eye Movement

The range of eye movement is not used specifically to diagnose diabetic retinopathy, but it is generally part of a comprehensive eye exam. Although the test for range of eye movement does not involve any high-tech equipment, it does give your eye care professional valuable information about the condition of your eye muscles and the nerves connected to them. Occasionally, diabetes may affect the nerves of the eye muscles and cause problems with eye movements. The eye doctor will test one eye first, then the other, and then the two eyes together. You will be asked to look upward, downward, and from side to side while the doctor holds an object in front of you and asks you to follow it with your eyes.

Testing for Distorted Vision

Your eye care specialist may check for any distortion or waviness in your vision by using the *Amsler grid*. This grid looks like a sheet of graph paper with a dark dot in the center. You will be asked to cover one eye and focus the open eye on the dot and say whether any of the lines on the grid appear wavy, distorted, blurry, or blank. If the answer is yes, it may be an indication of macular disease such as macular degeneration (damage to the macula in the center of the retina) or diabetic macular edema (swelling of the retina).

Amsler Grid

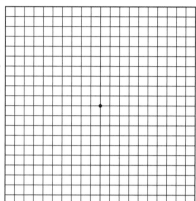

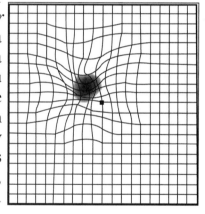

The Amsler grid is a test for checking yourself for symptoms of macular degeneration. The top grid represents normal vision. The bottom grid represents distortion of central vision, which is an early symptom of macular disease.

Dilation of the Pupils

For some parts of a comprehensive eye examination, your eye care specialist will likely use eyedrops to dilate, or widen, your pupils. Dilating the pupils provides the doctor with a better view of the internal structures of the eye—particularly the macula and the peripheral retina. It usually takes thirty minutes or more for the eyedrops to take full effect. After the pupils are fully dilated, the doctor may use a variety of sophisticated tools to examine the eye.

Dilation of the pupils often makes your vision blurred and your eyes sensitive to bright light. The effects of dilating eyedrops typically take about three to four hours to wear off. During this time, you may be more comfortable and see better if you wear sunglasses. Driving is not recommended after your pupils have been dilated.

Examination of the Front of the Eye

To examine the structures of the front of the eye, your eye care specialist will use a slit lamp. After you are seated comfortably with your chin in the chin support, the doctor will examine the parts of the front of the eye, including the following:

- *Eyelids:* The eyelids will be examined for any signs of infection or malfunction.
- *Conjunctiva:* This is the thin, transparent membrane that covers the white part of the eye as well as the inner surface of the eyelid. The doctor will check this area for evidence of inflammation, which can cause the white part of the eye to appear red and irritated.

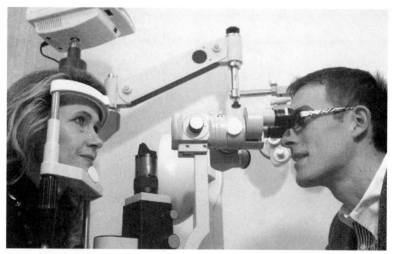

Eye care specialists use a slit lamp, with high-intensity light, to examine the inner structures of the eye.

When inflammation is present, it is often a sign of allergy or infection.

- *Cornea:* The cornea is the clear, dome-shaped front surface of the eye. It does most of the focusing work for the eye. When examining the cornea, the doctor will look for signs of inflammation, irritation, or infection.

- *Tear film:* The tear film is a protective liquid layer that lubricates the conjunctiva and the cornea. This film creates a smooth surface for light to pass through. With age, the tear film loses its ability to adequately lubricate the eye. This condition is referred to as *dry eyes syndrome.* Although dry eye is not a symptom of diabetic retinopathy, it may be irritating, and if it persists long term, it may be damaging to the health of the eye surface.

- *Iris:* The iris is the part of the eye that appears to have color. The iris controls the size of the pupil—reducing it in bright light and enlarging it in low light; this is the eye's way of regulating the amount of light coming into the eye. Your eye care specialist will check the appearance of the iris for growth of abnormal, tiny new vessels, which is a serious complication of severe proliferative diabetic retinopathy. This growth of tiny, fragile blood vessels is called *neovascularization.* Iris neovascularization can progress to a severe form of glaucoma called neovascular glaucoma.

- *Anterior chamber:* Separating the cornea and the iris is a clear, fluid-filled space called the anterior chamber. The doctor will check this area for signs of infection, inflammation, or hemorrhage.

- *Lens:* The eye's lens and cornea work together to focus images onto the retina. The doctor will check the lens for signs of clouding, which indicates the presence of a cataract. Because cataracts can significantly impair vision, it is important to check for this condition when you are experiencing vision problems. Individuals with diabetes are at higher risk than average for developing cataracts.

Examination of the Back of the Eye

Ophthalmoscopy allows your eye care specialist to view the structures at the back of the eye under magnification. Viewing the back of the eye is a critical part of your examination because the structures

---

Questions for Your Eye Care Specialist

- What type and stage of diabetic retinopathy do I have?

- Are both of my eyes affected at the same degree?

- How will I know if my diabetic retinopathy is progressing?

- What can I do to help manage my diabetic retinopathy?

- What kinds of treatments are available?

- Are there any symptoms I should watch for that might need immediate attention?

---

damaged by diabetic retinopathy are located in this area. The structures examined include the retina, choroid (layer of tissue that nourishes the back of the eye), blood vessels, optic disc (the point where the fibers of the optic nerve emerge from the eyeball), and vitreous.

There are two commonly used techniques for ophthalmoscopy. For the first technique, a doctor uses a slit lamp and a viewing lens to see a detailed, high-magnification examination of the macula and the optic nerve. The second technique, called *indirect ophthalmoscopy,* utilizes a special headset light and a handheld magnifier. Both these techniques allow examination of the following:

- *Vitreous gel:* This clear, jelly-like substance occupying the area between the lens and the retina is checked for signs of hemorrhage, inflammation, and liquefaction. *Liquefaction* occurs when the part of the vitreous gel turns to liquid—similar to melting Jello. Liquefaction can be the result of normal aging.

- *Optic nerve:* The optic nerve is like a cable that sends information from the eye to the brain. With diabetic retinopathy, abnormal blood vessels may grow over the optic nerve. This process, called neovascularization, refers to the abnormal development of tiny, leaky blood vessels in the eye. It is a sign of severe proliferative diabetic retinopathy.

- *Macula:* The macula is the center part of the retina and is critical for central vision. Because the macula can be subject to severe diabetic retinopathy damage, your doctor will pay special attention to this area during an exam. Specifically, the doctor will be looking for signs of blood, abnormal blood vessels, and thickening of tissue, indicating buildup of fluid (macular edema).

- *Peripheral retina:* This part of the retina outside the macula makes side vision possible. Diabetic retinopathy affects the entire retina, including the peripheral parts. Your eye care specialist will check it for signs of bleeding, growth of abnormal blood vessels, and retinal detachment.

Fundus Photography

Your doctor may take photographs of your retina to document the presence and severity of diabetic retinopathy. This is called *fundus photography*. The photographs are useful for future comparisons and evaluation of any progression of disease. The procedure is performed with a highly specialized camera that looks like a slit lamp. Your pupils may be dilated in order to obtain high-quality photographs of retinal periphery.

Fundus Fluorescein Angiography

Fundus fluorescein angiography is a special type of fundus photography that shows the blood circulation in the retina and choroid (the vessels that nourish the back of the eye). During this test an orange dye call fluorescein is injected into a vein in your arm. The dye travels through the bloodstream and, when it circulates through the retinal blood vessels, a special high-speed camera takes a series of photographs. These photos show the fine retinal blood vessels and the way the blood circulates through the retina. This allows your retina specialist to determine how much blood and fluid leakage may be present. The test also shows whether there are any areas of the retina that are not receiving blood and whether abnormal new blood vessels are forming.

Fundus fluorescein angiography is generally safe. You may notice yellow/orange discoloration of your skin and urine for one or two days after the test. Occasionally, you may feel nauseous within the first few minutes of injection of the dye, but this

Fundus Fluorescein Angiography

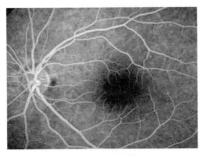

Normal eye as shown by fluorescein angiogram, a test that uses a special dye to examine the blood vessels of the retina.

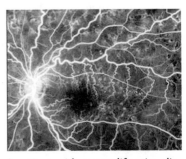

A patient with nonproliferative diabetic retinopathy shown here with fluorescein angiogram. The tiny white dots are abnormal dilations of retinal blood vessels called microaneurysms.

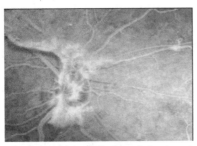

A patient with proliferative diabetic retinopathy has just received an injection of special dye. This fluorescein angiography shows abnormal growth of blood vessels at the optic disc.

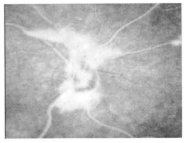

Same patient a few minutes after the injection of the dye. The fluorescein angiogram shows dye leaking from the abnormal new blood vessels.

passes quickly. Rarely, some individuals may have an allergic reaction to the fluorescein dye. This is more common if you have a history of multiple allergies. Kidney problems and renal dialysis are not affected by fluorescein angiography.

Anatomy of the Eye

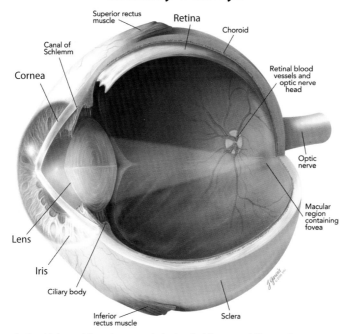

The retina is a thin layer of tissue that covers the back wall of the eye much like a wallpaper. It is sensitive to light and, through the optic nerve, it sends visual images to the brain. *Reprinted with permission. Copyright Thieme, 2009.*

Retina and Macula

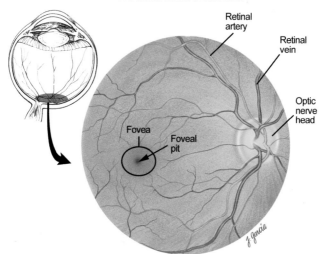

The macula is located toward the center of the retina. It is responsible for central vision and for seeing fine details and color. *Reprinted with permission. Copyright Thieme, 2009.*

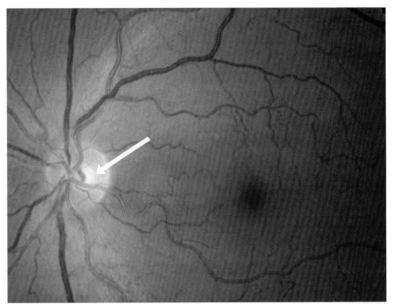

Normal retina. This retina shows healthy blood vessels and optic disc (indicated by the arrow). The optic disc is the point at which the optic nerve enters the retina.

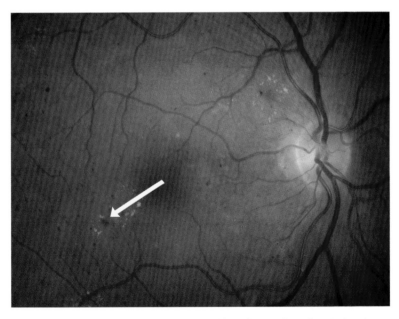

Mild non-proliferative diabetic retinopathy. Small red dots indicate tiny hemorrhages in the retina.

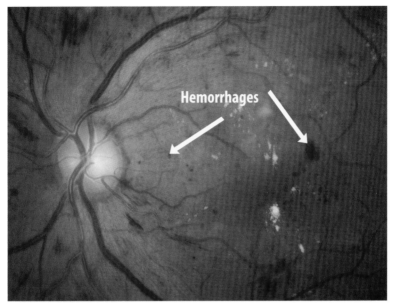

Severe nonproliferative diabetic retinopathy. Notice the presence of many hemorrhages (red dots) in this retina. Yellow spots are fatty deposits.

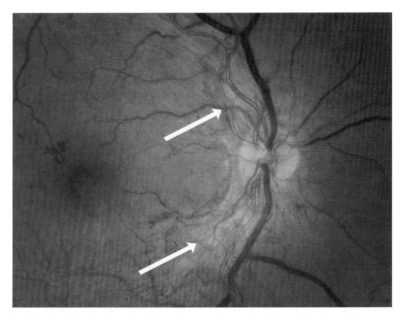

Proliferative diabetic retinopathy. Retina shows extensive growth of abnormal blood vessels (neovascularization) originating from the area of the optic disc.

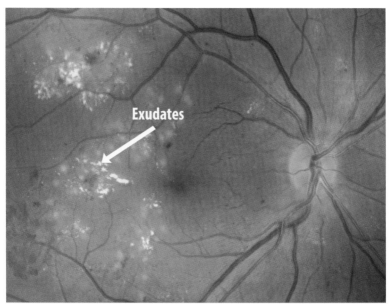

Diabetic macular edema. The yellow spots are fat deposits and indicate swelling (edema) of the macula.
Reprinted with permission. Copyright Thieme, 2009.

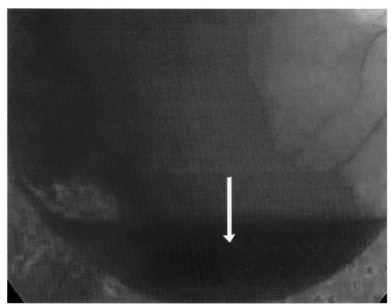

Vitreous hemorrhage. Bleeding into the vitreous gel has occurred as the result of severe proliferative diabetic retinopathy. The arrow points to the "boat-shaped" dark area in the lower eyeball that shows how the blood has accumulated. *Reprinted with permission. Copyright Thieme, 2009.*

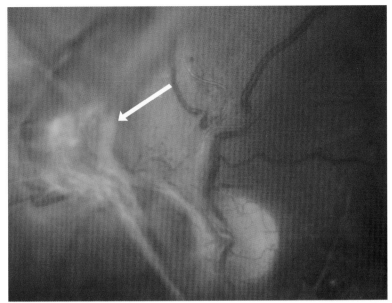

Tractional retinal detachment. The arrow shows where the retina has pulled away from the eye wall as the result of severe proliferative diabetic retinopathy.

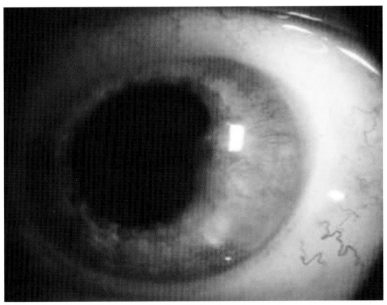

Neovascularization of iris. Severe proliferative diabetic retinopathy, showing growth of abnormal blood vessels (neovascularization) around the iris. This individual also has neovascular glaucoma, which is highly increased eye pressure. *Reprinted with permission. Copyright Thieme, 2009.*

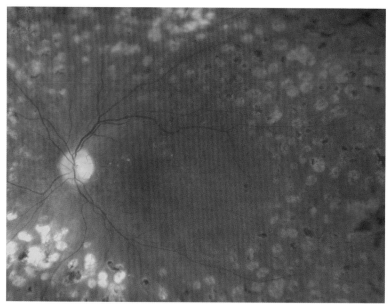

Panretinal laser photocoagulation. The yellow-grey spots are scars resulting from the laser treatment for abnormal blood vessels in the retina. Most laser scars do not affect vision.

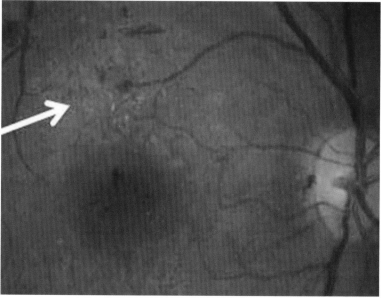

Laser photocoagulation. Old laser photocoagulation scars will darken as they heal and typically do not affect vision.

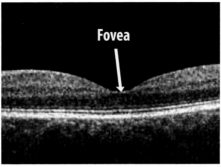

Optical coherence tomography (OCT). The top scan shows the smooth surface of a normal macula. The depression, the center of the macula, is normal. Below, the yellow in the scan's color map also represents a normal macula. The round numerical map, under the color map tells the ophthalmologist the thickness of the macula in micrometers.

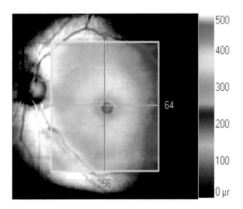

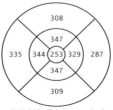

ILM-RPE Thickness (cm)

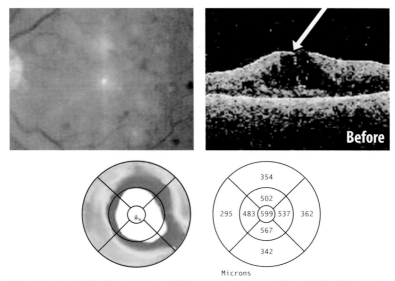

Before treatment. This OCT scan (above, right) shows macular edema, a buildup of fluid within the retina and macular tissues (arrow). The yellow and red in the color map represents the area of swelling.

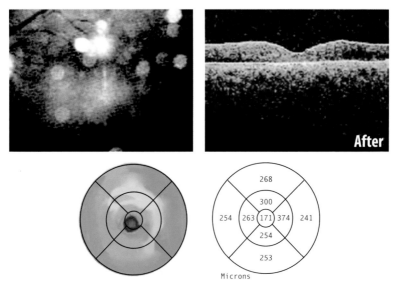

After treatment. The OCT scan (above, right) shows a smoother macula and the color map's greens and yellows represent resolution of macular edema (swelling).

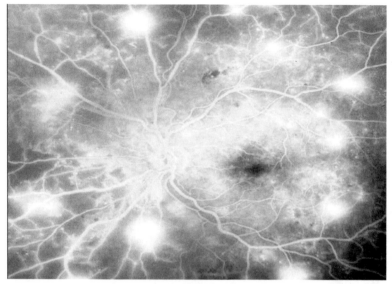

A fluorescein angiogram of a patient with proliferative diabetic retinopathy shows patchy white areas, which are leaking abnormal blood vessels in the retina.

Optical Coherence Tomography

Optical coherence tomography (OCT) is a noninvasive test that is commonly performed when macular problems are suspected. The test uses light technology to produce a high-resolution scan of the macula. It is not an X-ray, but it shows a cross-sectional image of the retina that allows a doctor to measure its thickness; this permits the doctor to see if the shape of the macula is normal or abnormal. The doctor can also identify the presence of fluid to determine if leakage has resulted in the buildup of fluid under the macula or within the retina. Optical coherence tomography is an excellent tool for diagnosing and monitoring most macular diseases including diabetic macular edema and macular degeneration.

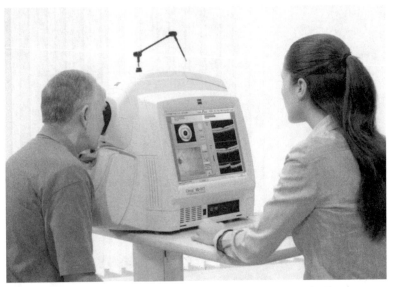

Optical coherence tomography (OCT) is like a CT scan of the macula. The scan uses light technology to map changes in the macula. *Photo courtesy of Carl Zeiss Meditec, Inc.*

The device used for this test is similar to a slit lamp. A technician will ask you to place your chin in a chin rest and look straight into the machine as it takes the scan. The evaluation takes about fifteen minutes.

B-Scan Ultrasonography

Your eye specialist may order *B-scan ultrasonography* to view your retina. Using high-frequency sound waves to build a picture, this test is similar to a sonogram that OB/GYN doctors use to evaluate a fetus during pregnancy. This B-scan ultrasonography is helpful when bleeding or hemorrhaging in the vitreous gel, severe corneal problems, or cataract prevent your doctor from seeing the back of your eye. The ultrasound is a painless and relatively quick office

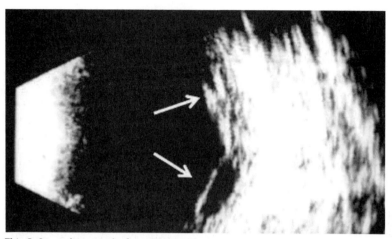

This B-Scan ultrasound of a patient with severe proliferative diabetic retinopathy shows a tractional retinal detachment. The arrows show the retina has pulled away from the eye wall.

exam. It is performed while you are seated or lying down with your eyes closed. After a gel is placed on your eyelids, the doctor navigates the B-scan probe gently over the eyelids. The test is helpful in checking for retinal tears or detachments. B-scan ultrasonography does not have any known side effects on the eye.

After Your Diagnosis

Any diagnosis involving potential loss of vision can be worrying. It is frightening to think how your life and independence might be affected if you cannot see well. Diabetic retinopathy is a serious condition, but you can take steps to protect your vision. The key is to control your diabetes and undergo comprehensive eye examinations at regular intervals to detect and treat problems before they become serious.

In Summary

Because diabetic retinopathy can occur in both type 1 and type 2 diabetes, you must undergo an initial comprehensive eye examination after either diagnosis.

- A thorough retina evaluation involves reviewing the medical history, basic vision and eye pressure measurements, and dilation of the pupil for a detailed retinal examination. In addition, a variety of tests may be performed to determine the severity of the retinopathy and presence of serious sight-threatening conditions such as macular edema (swelling or thickening of macula) and abnormal new vessels (neovascularization). These tests include fundus photography, fundus fluorescein angiography, optical coherence tomography (OCT), and B-scan ultrasonography. The visit to your retina specialist may last two or more hours, depending on the tests and treatments that may be necessary.

- Diabetic retinopathy is classified either as nonproliferative diabetic retinopathy, the less severe form of the disease, or proliferative diabetic retinopathy, the advanced form of the disease.

- Your eye specialist may recommend evaluation and possible treatment at various intervals depending on the changes in your eyes and the stage of the disease.

3   Treatment for Nonproliferative Diabetic Retinopathy

You'll recall that nonproliferative diabetic retinopathy is the milder form of retinopathy. Treatment is generally not needed for mild, moderate, and even severe nonproliferative diabetic retinopathy.

It is crucial that you manage your diabetes carefully, as well as undergo comprehensive eye exams at least once a year or at shorter intervals if significant retinal and macular changes are occurring.

Treatment for Macular Edema

If you have nonproliferative diabetic retinopathy, and you develop macular edema, you will need treatment to avoid vision loss. You may need multiple treatment sessions that includes eye injections, called intravitreal injections; you may also need, retinal laser photocoagulation, which involves stabilizing the tissues with a laser beam.

Intravitreal injections are a powerful tool for treating several retinal diseases, including macular edema. If you have this swelling of the macula, your doctor may suggest injections of medication in the eye to slow the leakage of blood vessels and reduce swell-

Intravitreal Injection

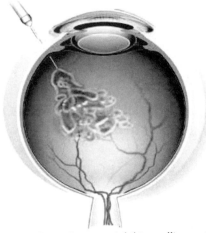

Medications may be injected into the eye to inhibit swelling and leaking of blood vessels. The eye is anesthetized prior to injection. Most patients report no major pain during the injection.

ing. Because the eye is numbed, most patients do not find the injections painful. Your doctor may choose from several types of medications to inject.

Intravitrial Injections

One of the injections used to treat macular edema involves the use of *anti-vascular endothelial growth factor (anti-VEGF) drugs.* To understand how these drugs work, note that a special protein is produced by the damaged retina that promotes leakage from existing retinal blood vessels; this, in turn, causes the macula to swell. The anti-VEGF agents target this protein, reducing the leakage, and allowing the macular swelling to subside.

Although anti-VEGF drugs are effective in the treatment of diabetic retinopathy, they were developed initially to treat cancer. You may wonder why a drug used to treat cancer is being used to treat diabetic retinopathy. The drugs inhibit the abnormal growth and leakage of blood vessels. Because cancer cells need abnormal blood vessels to flourish, scientists rightly believed that starving those cells of their blood source could reduce tumor growth.

Scientists discovered that in much smaller doses these drugs are an excellent treatment for certain eye diseases, including diabetic retinopathy, in which the underlying problem is leaky blood vessels. For example, clinical studies have shown that the anti-VEGF drug Avastin *(bevacizumab)* is an effective treatment for diabetic retinopathy, even though it was originally developed for the treatment of colon cancer.

Because the Food and Drug Administration (FDA) has yet to officially authorize Avastin for the treatment of any eye disease, it is currently being used as what's referred to as "off-label usage" for the treatment of diabetic retinopathy. That means your doctor is prescribing the drug for a condition other than the disease for which it was originally approved. Patients should rest assured, however, knowing that "off-label" drug usage is a common and safe practice.

Your eye specialist also may recommend another drug, Lucentis *(ranibizumab),* which is similar to Avastin. Lucentis is FDA-approved for treatment of macular edema caused by diabetes. Numerous clinical studies have shown the safety and effectiveness of Lucentis.

Injections with VEGF-Trap Drugs

Another group of drugs called vascular endothelial growth factor-trap (VEGF-trap) are similar to the anti-VEGF drugs. These drugs, which attack the growth of abnormal blood vessels and also reduce leakage from damaged blood vessels, were originally approved for the treatment of wet macular degeneration. One specific drug, called Eylea *(aflibercept)*, has shown promising results for treating diabetic macular edema and will likely be approved in the near future.

Injections with Steroids

As another treatment option, your doctor may recommend steroid injections. These medications make retinal blood vessels less leaky by working on the cells that line the vessels. In a normal eye, there is no excess fluid leakage. With diabetes, however, gaps between cells may behave like sieves. So, by tightening these gaps, steroid medications reduce the leakage of the fluid into the retina, allowing the macular edema to resolve with time.

Steroid medications such as Kenalog *(triamcinolone acetonide)*, Triesence *(preservative-free triamcinolone acetonide)*, and Ozurdex *(dexamethasone)* are not FDA-labeled for diabetic retinopathy. They are used as "off-label" treatments. They are often recommended as second-line agents or in addition to anti-VEGF drugs for treatment of diabetic macular edema.

Ozurdex is a slow-release form of *dexamethasone,* which is a potent steroid. Ozurdex comes in the form of a small pellet that is implanted into the vitreous cavity by an injection in the doctor's office. The effect of the medication usually lasts three to four months. During this period you may notice one or more floaters usually in the shape of "bars" or "cylinders." Ozurdex is approved for the treatment of macular edema that may occur as a result of retinal vein occlusion, blockage of small vessels that carry blood away from the retina.

Currently, the use if this medication for treating diabetic macular edema is considered "off-label," meaning it has not been approved by the FDA. It will, howver, likely be approved in the future.

Another slow-release steriod implant called Iluvien *(fluocinoloneacetonide)* is under consideration for approval by the FDA. This drug is used to treat chronic diabetic macular edema that does not respond to other treatments. The Iluvien implant lasts one to two years and has already been approved for use in Europe.

Your eye specialist will discuss which drug is appropriate for you, how often it will be administered, and how it might be used in conjunction with other treatments.

Receiving an Eye Injection

An injection procedure is performed in a doctor's office. Usually, one eye is treated at a time; however, sometimes both eyes are treated. Prior to the injection, your eye will be numbed and cleansed. The antiseptic or cleansing solution may cause a temporary burning sensation. Various techniques are used to anesthetize the eye, including numbing eyedrops or gel and an injectable anesthetic, similar to what you would receive in a dentist's office.

The eye specialist will use a small device, called an *eyelid speculum,* to help keep your eyelids open during the injection. You may be asked to look in a specific direction as your retina specialist inserts a tiny needle into the white of the eye. Most patients do not find this injection painful. It is over in seconds.

Your doctor may or may not suggest an eye patch or antibiotic eyedrops for a few days following the procedure. Ideally, you should have someone drive you home because you may experience temporary light sensitivity and blurring in the eye that had the injection.

Whether you are receiving anti-VEGF or steroid injections, you will be revaluated in one or two months to monitor the response to the treatment and to see if further treatment is needed. Because diabetes is a chronic condition that continues to damage the retina, problems such as macular edema or the abnormal growth of tiny new vessels (neovascularization) can return and require additional treatments. It is important to control your diabetes and see your eye specialist regularly to catch any recurrence before it causes irreversible damage.

Potential Side Effects of Eye Injections

Side effects produced by intravitreal injections are generally localized and minimal. You may experience:

- mild irritation such as a gritty or scratchy sensation in the eye. The irritation usually resolves in a few days.

- tearing, bloodstained tears, floaters, and even hemorrhages in the white of the eye. These symptoms usually fade away in a few days or weeks, causing no visual effects.

- burning and irritation of the treated eye. This is a common reaction caused by irritation of povidone-iodine (a disinfecting solution) that typically lasts less than a day. You may also develop minor scratches of the eye surface. If your symptoms do not clear up within a day, call your eye specialist.

- infections, inflammation, increased eye pressure, vitreous hemorrhage, or retinal tear and detachment. These serious complications occur very rarely.

Additional effects of steroid injections include progression of an existing cataract as well as increased eye pressure. However, in most cases the increase in eye pressure can be alleviated with eyedrops until the effect of the medication wears off. Some of the steroid medications may result in floaters or "floating clouds" in the visual field. Fortunately, this effect is temporary and improves over a period of a few weeks.

Potential Complications of Eye Injections

Eye injections are considered safe procedures, and complications are rare. The injections are not without potential risks, however. The injections may cause vitreous hemorrhage, retinal tear, retinal detachment, or infection.

Focal Laser Photocoagulation

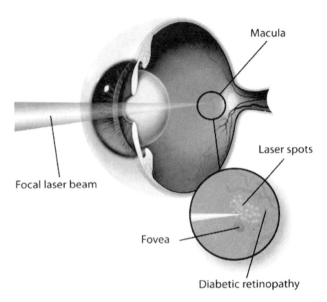

Macula

Laser spots

Focal laser beam

Fovea

Diabetic retinopathy

During focal laser photocoagulation, tiny bursts of laser light penetrate the eye to treat leaking blood vessels of the retina.

You may have heard that high doses of anti-VEGF or VEGF-trap medications given intravenously for treatment of some cancers my be linked to increased problems such as high blood pressure, heart attack, and stroke. Because treatment of macular edema involves only tiny doses of these medications, it is unlikely for these intravitreal injections to cause other health issues.

Focal Laser Photocoagulation
for Macular Edema

A laser procedure, called *focal laser photocoagulation,* is a common treatment for leaky blood vessels in the macular region of the retina. This treatment uses laser

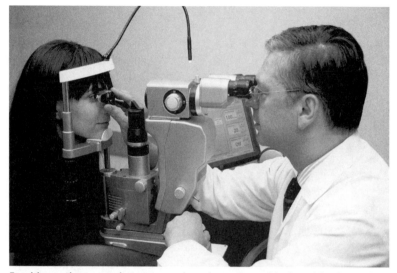

Focal laser photocoagulation uses a laser beam to seal leaking blood vessels to reduce vision loss. During a treatment, a physician directs tiny bursts of laser light into the eye.

light to reduce leakage, promote absorption, and reduce vision loss. Your doctor will recommend the procedure if fluid has accumulated under the macula, causing it to swell. At one time, focal laser photocoagulation was the main treatment for diabetic macular edema. Over the past decade, however, the injectable drugs have offered additional treatment options. Depending on the type, severity, and location of macular edema, your retina specialist may recommend laser treatment, injections, or both.

Undergoing Focal Laser Photocoagulation for Macula Edema

This procedure is performed in the doctor's office. You will be seated at a slit lamp, an instrument that allows the retina specialist to see the retina and other

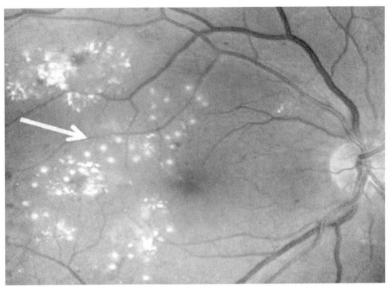

This photograph was taken few minutes after a focal laser photocoagulation treatment in a patient with diabetic macular edema (swelling). The white spots are tiny marks made by the laser. *Reprinted with permission. Copyright Thieme, 2009.*

structures in the back of the eye. You'll rest your chin and forehead on supports. Numbing eyedrops will be placed in your eye. After the eye is numb, a special lens will be placed on the surface of the eye. The lens allows your doctor to clearly see the retina and macula, allowing him or her to target the area for laser treatment.

The slit lamp used for laser photocoagulation is specially modified to allow the physician to see the retina and deliver the laser light. The laser light is focused and very short flashes are directed at the retina. Usually, about fifty to one hundred laser spots, each about the size of a fine-tip pen point, are administered to the area. Focal laser photocoagulation usually takes one session. Although the actual procedure

---

**Management of Nonproliferative
Diabetic Retinopathy**

- Maintain general health
- Control diabetes, body weight, blood pressure, and
  lipids
- Exercise
- Stop smoking
- Schedule regular retina evaluations
- Receive treatment for macular edema if present
  —Intravitreal injections
  —Focal laser photocoagulation

---

may take about ten minutes, it may take one or two hours to prepare you, particularly if more tests are necessary prior to the procedure. If both eyes are involved, each eye is treated separately at least a few days part. The laser treatment may take a few months to take effect.

Potential Side Effects of
Focal Laser Photocoagulation

Focal laser photocoagulation is not painful and patients usually tolerate it well. Most patients have no adverse side effects. In rare instances, individuals notice light, dark, or blank spots in their visual field. These spots are so tiny that they are not bothersome, and they usually fade away within a few months.

Potential Complications of
Focal Laser Photocoagulation

It is possible, but rare, for laser photocoagulation to cause some vision loss. Still, patients with significant macular edema will benefit more by having the procedure than not having it.

In Summary

- Treatment for nonproliferative diabetic retinopathy is usually not required.

- One of the complications that may develop with nonproliferative diabetic retinopathy is macular edema, swelling of the macula.

- Treatments for macular edema include injectable medications and laser procedures.

- How well treatments may work depends on the severity of changes in the eye and the type of vision problems you have.

- Early detection of retinopathy and treatment is the key to maintaining good eyesight and preventing permanent damage.

Treatments for Proliferative Diabetic Retinopathy

4

The treatment goal for proliferative diabetic retinopathy is to stop damage to the retina before it causes irreversible vision loss. Even though doctors may not be able to cure the disease or fully reverse damage that has already occurred, they have treatments to slow the progression of diabetic retinopathy and help preserve your existing sight.

Because the effects of proliferative diabetic retinopathy are unique to each person, your eye specialist will adapt various therapies to fit your needs. He or she may choose from any of the following treatments:

- *Panretinal laser photocoagulation,* which is a laser treatment that slows or stops growth of abnormal blood vessels.

- *Injections of drugs into the eye* to inhibit the growth of abnormal blood vessels and also reduce leakage.

- *Vitrectomy,* a special eye surgery, that is used to treat complications of severe proliferative diabetic retinopathy such as bleeding into the vitreous gel, retinal detachment, and severe macular edema that does not respond to other forms of treatment.

Panretinal Laser Photocoagulation

The first line of treatment for stopping or slowing damage to the retina due to proliferative diabetic retinopathy is *panretinal laser photocoagulation (PRP)*. It utilizes split-second bursts of high-energy laser light to halt the growth of abnormal new vessels.

The procedure is also commonly referred to "scatter" retinal laser photocoagulation.

Note that this laser treatment works best for fragile, new blood vessels before they start to bleed. The sooner the problem is recognized, the more effective the treatment is and the better the outcome. For example, once bleeding has occurred in the vitreous gel, the ability to perform laser treatments is compromised.

For a panretinal laser photocoagulation treatment, your doctor will apply sharply focused laser beams, the size of pencil points. As many as 2,000 spots may be applied to the peripheral retina. During the treatment, you may feel some discomfort or pain because of the high intensity of the laser. Because a large number of laser spots are necessary to address widespread abnormal vessel growth, you may have to undergo a second treatment session. You may also need additional treatments later because diabetic retinopathy is a chronic problem that continues to damage the retina, especially if your diabetes is not well controlled.

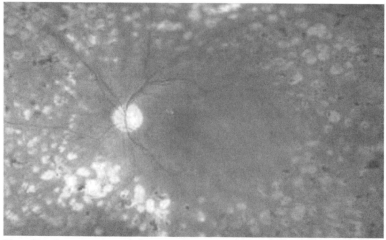

The white dots are tiny scars from panretinal laser photocoagulation, used to stop the growth of abnormal blood vessels. The procedure is intended to reduce loss of vision.

Undergoing Panretinal Laser Photocoagulation

Panretinal laser photocoagulation is an outpatient office procedure. First, your pupil will be dilated. After the dilation eyedrops are inserted, it takes thirty to forty-five minutes for the pupils to become dilated. The actual laser procedure takes about fifteen minutes.

The procedure for panretinal laser photocoagulation is similar to that for a focal laser photocoagulation. You will be seated in front of the laser device with your forehead and chin in supports. Because it is important to remain still, you will likely be given a target to stare at with your other eye. You may see flashes as the laser beam burns tiny spots on the retina. Your doctor will carefully avoid the optic nerve and the macula. Laser photocoagulation is well tolerated by most people; you may, however, feel a temporary discomfort with each burst of the laser. Results from the treatment are usually evident in about two months.

After your treatment, you may or may not require medications to reduce any inflammation. Most patients do not need pain relievers because discomfort is typically minimal. You may want to wear sunglasses and ask a friend to drive you home after the procedure because the medication to dilate your pupils will take several hours to wear off. In the meantime, your eyes will be sensitive to sunlight. Most patients can return to normal activity within a day with no restrictions.

Potential Side Effects of Panretinal Laser Photocoagulation

Side effects that can occur with panretinal laser photocoagulation may include:

- burning sensation and eye irritation caused by the contact lens the doctor uses to see the retina. The discomfort, however, is not severe and usually clears up in a day.
- blurriness and difficulty in focusing on near objects. This usually resolves within a few weeks.
- minor visual disturbances, such as visual spots or blanks. They either fade over time or are so miniscule that they won't interfere with your eyesight.
- a decrease in peripheral, night, and even color vision. The reductions, however, are usually slight and occur only if extensive PRP is required.

Potential Complications of
Panretinal Laser Photocoagulation

Serious complications of panretinal laser photocoagulation are rare. Potential side-effects include increase in macular edema, transient eye inflammation, vitreous hemorrhage, retinal detachment, inadvertent burns to the macula, diminished night vision, or diminished peripheral (side) vision.

Injections for Proliferative Diabetic Retinopathy

The intravitreal injections of anti-VEGF drugs used to treat macular edema are also used to treat proliferative diabetic retinopathy. The injections are often used in combination with panretinal laser photocoagulation.

As explained in the previous chapter, anti-VEGF drugs are based on the idea that abnormal blood vessels thrive because a special stimulating protein, called vascular endothelial growth factor (VEGF), promotes their growth. The anti-VEGF drugs target this factor in such a way that vessels stabilize, stop leaking, and shrink.

Currently, the first line treatment for proliferative diabetic retinopathy is panretinal laser photocoagulation. Anti-VEGF drugs are useful additions in cases of severe proliferative diabetic retinopathy or in cases with vitreous hemorrhage interfering with laser treatment. In the later situation, treatment with anti-VEGF drugs temporarily stabilizes the abnormal blood vessels that are bleeding, allowing the vitreous hemorrhage to get absorbed. Once the vitreous hemorrhage clears, panretinal laser photocoagulation can be performed.

Management of Proliferative Diabetic Retinopathy

- Maintain general health
- Control diabetes, body weight, blood pressure, and lipids
- Exercise
- Stop smoking
- Schedule regular retina evaluations
- Undergo panretinal laser photocoagulation
- Receive treatment of vitreous hemorrhage if present
  —Intravitreal injections
  —Panretinal laser photocoagulation
  —Vitrectomy surgery

Injections for Macular Edema

As mentioned in earlier, diabetic macular edema (swelling in the center of the retina) may occur in either type of diabetic retinopathy, but is more common among those with proliferative diabetic retinopathy. As mentioned in the previous chapter, treatment for macular edema typically involves injections that reduce leakage of blood vessels, which reduces swelling. Depending on the severity of the macular edema, your retina specialist may also use laser treatments to stop the leakage from tiny blood vessels in the eye.

Potential Side Effects of Injections

Side effects of anti-VEGF injections for treatment of proliferative diabetic retinopathy are generally mild and similar to those discussed in the section for the treatment of macular edema. Irritation, burning sensation, and a "blood-shot" eye are the most common side effects that resolve spontaneously after a few days. One uncommon side effect of anti-VEGF injections for proliferative diabetic retinopathy is an increase in vitreous pulling on the retina leading to the progression of a tractional retinal detachment; if this occurs, it is usually mild and does not cause serious problems.

Potential Complications of Injections

As explained earlier, eye injections for diabetic retinopathy are considered safe procedures; they do, however, carry potential risks such as vitreous hemorrhage, retinal tear, retinal detachment, and infection.

Treatment for Vitreous Hemorrhage

Vitreous hemorrhage is a common complication of untreated proliferative diabetic retinopathy. As you may recall, a vitreous hemorrhage involves bleeding into the vitreous, the clear gel in the center of the eyeball. This condition initially starts with the onset of floaters if the hemorrhage is mild. Severe vitreous hemorrhage causes sudden, painless loss of vision.

A vitreous hemorrhage not only affects the patient's vision, but it also obscures the physician's view of the retina during an examination. Sometimes the vitreous hemorrhage is so severe that your eye doctor may not be able to see the retina at all. In this situation, an ultrasound scan is a useful tool that allows the doctor to evaluate the retina for any retinal detachment behind the vitreous hemorrhage. Vitreous hemorrhage also prevents delivery of laser treatment to the retina as the blood blocks the laser light from reaching the retina.

The initial treatment for vitreous hemorrhage often includes a period of reduced physical activity and observation to allow for the hemorrhage to be absorbed by the eye. Injections of anti-VGF drugs may be used to temporarily stabilize the abnormal blood vessels until the vitreous blood clears enough for panretinal laser photocoagulation to be performed.

You may be asked to use multiple pillows to elevate your head while you are sleeping. Gravity will help settle vitreous hemorrhage to the lower portion of your eye, improving your vision during the day.

Vitrectomy: Surgery for Vitreous Hemorrhage

In cases of severe vitreous hemorrhage or when the hemorrhage does not clear spontaneously, surgery to remove the vitreous hemorrhage may be recommended by your retina specialist. The surgical procedure is called a vitrectomy. It is a microsurgical technique to remove the vitreous gel core of your eye. The gel is typically replaced with a solution similar to the natural eye fluid. In these situations, vitrectomy improves vision and also makes it possible for the surgeon to better assess the retina to determine if further treatment is needed. In some cases, additional laser photocoagulation may be performed during vitrectomy.

Vitrectomy

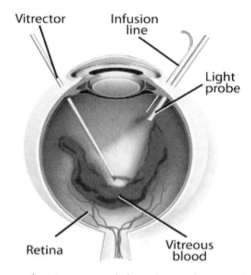

During a vitrectomy, a physician inserts a light probe into the eye and then uses a cutting tool to remove the vitreous gel. The eye may be filled with gas or oil to hold the retina in place during healing.

Undergoing a Vitrectomy

If you are undergoing a vitrectomy, your procedure will usually be performed in an outpatient setting under local anesthesia. You will also be given medication to lightly sedate you, and you will not feel any pain.

Using high magnification provided by a special operating microscope, the retina surgeon will make three tiny incisions in the white part of the eye. The incisions are used to pass delicate instruments into the eye, beginning with a light probe. This illuminates the inside of the eye including the vitreous and retina. Then, with a special, controlled cutting device, the vitreous gel is removed along with any scar tissue,

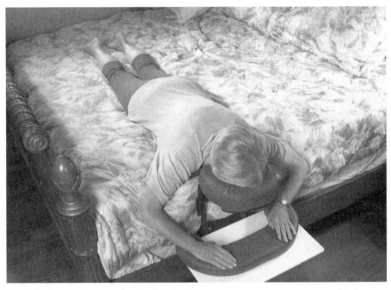

Vitrectomy patients who've had a gas or silicone bubble injected to hold the retina in place are required to keep their heads in a face-down position for several days after the surgery. Most patients are allowed a ten-minute break each hour.
Photo courtesy of Comfort Solutions / www.facedownsolutions.com

abnormal vessels, and blood clots. As the gel is being removed, a solution is infused simultaneously through the third incision to maintain pressure in the eye and prevent it from collapsing. If the retina is torn or detached, either a gas bubble or silicone oil bubble is injected into the eye at the end of the surgery; this holds the retina in place until the laser treatment takes effect.

Vitrectomy surgery may take between thirty minutes and three hours, depending on the complexity of the case. Most patients go home the same day of the procedure. You will likely need to wear an eye shield to protect the eye, especially during sleeping and showering.

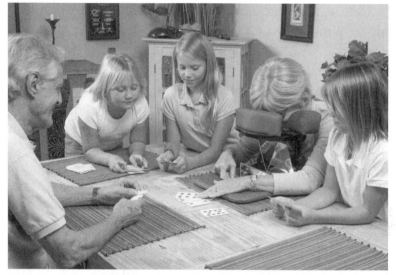

Special headrests may be rented or purchased by vitrectomy patients who are required to keep their heads facing down after their surgery.
Photo courtesy of Comfort Solutions / www.facedownsolutions.com

After surgery your eyelids and the eye may
appear swollen, red, or bruised. You will need anti-
inflammatory and antibiotic eye drops after the surgery
to reduce inflammation and the risk of infection. The
redness usually fades after several weeks. You may
or may not need pain medication, depending on the
extent of your surgery. If a gas bubble has been used,
you will not be able to travel by airplane or to higher
altitudes; your vision will be blurred until the bubble
is absorbed and is replaced by eye fluid.

Potential Complications of Vitrectomy

There are potential risks associated with a
vitrectomy surgery. The most common complication is
development of cataract or progression of an existing
cataract. This is not considered a serious complication

and can be taken care of by cataract surgery. If you already have had cataract surgery, this is not an issue. The procedure may cause transient elevated pressure inside the eye, especially in individuals who have glaucoma. Other potential risks include additional bleeding into the vitreous space, retinal detachment, and infection. Your retina specialist will monitor you closely for any signs of such complications.

Restrictions after Vitrectomy

After a vitrectomy, you will be given specific instructions. Too much moving about may damage the healing, delicate tissues in your eye. Restrictions will include no bending, heavy lifting, or exercise in the immediate days following a vitrectomy.

If you had a gas or silicone bubble injected into your eye to treat a torn or detached retina, your doctor will give you additional special instructions for positioning your head. For several days after the surgery, you will need to keep your head positioned so that you are facing down or looking down. This positioning allows the gas or oil bubble to hold the retina in place while it heals.

Face-down positioning is a tedious task, and your doctor may allow you to take a ten-minute break every hour. You cannot sleep on your back; you must sleep on your stomach with your head slightly tilted to the side. Your retina specialist may recommend a special device to support your head for sleeping face-down at night; placing extra pillows around you will help prevent you from rolling over as you sleep. You will likely also be instructed to keep your head positioned downward during the day, during your waking hours. Your doctor may recommend another device that cradles your head in the correct position for use during the day.

Depending on which type of gas is used, it may take two to eight weeks for the gas bubble to be absorbed and replaced by your natural eye fluid. Your vision will be blurred until the gas bubble is absorbed. If you have received an injection of silicone oil rather than a gas bubble, however, note that silicone oil does not get absorbed. It stays in the vitreous cavity until it is removed with a minor surgical procedure three or four months after the initial surgery. You will need avoid sleeping on your back as long as the silicone oil remains inside your eye.

In addition, if you have received a gas bubble, air travel or going to high altitude locations are strictly prohibited. The reduced atmospheric pressure of high altitudes can cause a bubble to expand, which may trigger dangerously elevated eye pressure. Your doctor will tell you when it is safe to travel by air. If you had a silicone oil injection in your eye, high altitudes and air travel are permitted.

Vitrectomy for Other Types of Retinal Damage

Your eye specialist may use vitrectomy surgery to repair other damage caused by diabetic retinopathy. This procedure is commonly used to treat other disorders such as tractional retinal detachment, epiretinal membrane, and neovascular glaucoma.

Tractional Retinal Detachment

As explained in an earlier chapter, tractional retinal detachment occurs when abnormal new blood vessels and scar tissue grow along the surface of the retina and attach firmly to the back of the vitreous gel. The retina and this gel are tightly bound, so when the abnormal blood vessels and the scar tissue contract and the vitreous pulls away, it exerts traction on the retina. This causes the retina to separate from the back of the eye.

With severe traction, the retina can tear, leading to a more serious from of detachment called *rhegmatagenous retinal detachment.* If this occurs, you will likely see shadows or large dark areas in your vision. If the macula is involved, there will be severe vision loss.

Many tractional retinal detachments that are away from the macula region do not require surgery. If the macula is involved or is endangered, however, vitrectomy is recommended to reduce risk of further vision loss. Removing the vitreous with surgery releases the traction so it no longer pulls on the retina and allows it to reattach. Laser photocoagulation may also be used at the time of vitrectomy to reduce growth of abnormal vessels or to treat retinal tears. Again, after a vitrectomy you will need to remain inactive for several days, according to your doctor's instructions.

Epiretinal Membrane

An *epiretinal membrane* is an abnormal wrinkling that occurs when a thin fibrous sheet grows on the inner surface of the retina in the macular region. Sometimes it develops as a healing response to various eye conditions such as retinal tears and retinal detachment. Because the epiretinal membrane is firmly attached to the underlying macula, as it contracts it causes the retina to wrinkle. Usually, there is no visual impact, unless the membrane distorts and wrinkles the macula significantly. In these cases the central vision becomes blurred and distorted.

If an epiretinal membrane is interfering significantly with your sight, your retina surgeon will perform vitrectomy surgery in conjunction with a "membrane peel." After removing the vitreous, fine forceps are used to gently peel away the membrane. Tiny stitches may be used to close the incisions. The same procedure may be used to remove the internal limiting membrane, a naturally occurring tissue in front of the macula. Eliminating this membrane may reduce macular swelling (macular edema) that is resistant to other treatments.

Neovascular Glaucoma

A severe form of glaucoma, *neovascular glaucoma* may sometimes be treated in the same way chronic open-angle glaucoma is treated. In some cases, however, vitrectomy may be required.

In this case, the goal of the vitrectomy is to allow the retina specialist to use a special laser to reduce the VEGF load. *VEGF* refers to the vascular endothelial growth factor; it is a protein is normally present in every person. It allows such things as healing of wounds, clot prevention, bone growth, and healing. This protein, however, is sometimes unregulated in people with diabetic retinopathy and it causes leakage of serum from normal retinal capillaries causing diabetic macular edema (swelling). Or it can cause new blood vessel formation on the retina or the iris.

By performing the vitrectomy to remove the gel in the middle of the eye, the physician can then use the laser to stop the abnormal "supply" of the protein VEGF. This can stop further vision loss from occurring.

Follow-Up Care

After the proliferative diabetic retinopathy is brought under control, you will be evaluated by your retina specialist at approximately four-month intervals. This will allow early detection and treatment of any recurring disease activity. Detecting the damage when it is still in the early stages can preserve your remaining eyesight. Otherwise, if left untreated, most individuals with severe proliferative diabetic retinopathy will lose their sight.

Treatment for Other Eye Diseases Associated with Diabetes

Individuals with diabetic retinopathy are at risk for other eye problems that may require treatment. These problems include glaucoma, cataracts, optic neuropathy, retinal vein occlusion, and corneal problems.

Glaucoma

Individuals with diabetes have a higher chance of developing *chronic open-angle glaucoma*. In this condition, the pressure inside the eye rises above normal and, with time, damages the optic nerve. This results in loss of peripheral vision, which if not treated, may progress to loss of central vision also.

Treatment for glaucoma may include pressure-lowering eye drops, laser treatment of the drainage angle of the eye, and in some cases, surgery. Glaucoma surgery involves making a tunnel into the front compartment of the eye or placing a drainage tube in the eye. Those with glaucoma should be monitored with require regular evaluations of eye pressure, the optic disc, and visual field testing. These examinations are performed by a general ophthalmologist or a glaucoma specialist.

Neovascular glaucoma is a severe form of glaucoma that is most commonly associated with advance diabetic eye disease. Treatment of neovascular glaucoma is often the same as for chronic open-angle glaucoma, but as noted earlier, it also sometimes requires surgery—a vitrectomy.

Cataracts

Individuals with diabetes are more prone to developing cataracts. Cataracts in diabetics develop at a younger age and sometimes more severely compared to nondiabetic individuals. Cataract surgery may be considered once the cataract is severe enough to reduce vision to the point of interfering with daily tasks. With today's surgical techniques, cataracts can be treated effectively. If you have active proliferative diabetic retinopathy or macular edema, however, your doctor may delay cataract surgery until the retinopathy is more stable. The exception is if the cataract is preventing evaluation or treatment of the retina.

During cataract surgery, the natural lens is removed and a new, artificial lens is inserted. The new lens is called an *intraocular lens (IOL)*. Prior to cataract surgery, you will undergo an ultrasound to measure the size and shape of your eye to determine the correct strength of the artificial intraocular lens that will be implanted.

Cataract surgery is typically performed on an outpatient basis. You will likely be awake for the procedure; your eye will be numbed and you will receive medicine intravenously to help you relax. After you are sedated, your doctor will make a small incision in the eye and remove the cloudy lens (the cataract) with a process called *phacoemulsification;* this procedure breaks the cataract into small pieces with a special probe that moves with a frequency similar to that of an ultrasound. After the cataract is broken up, the metal probe extracts the pieces like a vacuum.

Then, an artificial intraocular lens is positioned within the capsule, the cellophane-like wrapping surrounding the original lens. Although the front portion of the capsule has been removed, the back portion is left to support the lens implant.

Some patients develop what is called an "after-cataract" following the surgery. This is a clouding of the remaining lens capsule. Although it can be part of normal healing, it also can interfere with vision. If needed, your doctor will use a special laser to create an opening in the capsule that allows light to pass through to the retina. This procedure, called *posterior capsulotomy*, is a painless and quick in-office procedure that often improves the vision.

Cataract surgery is usually successful. Even with an excellent outcome, however, your vision may still be affected by your diabetic retinopathy.

Optic Neuropathy

The optic nerve carries images from the eye to the brain. *Optic neuropathy* occurs when the optic nerve is receiving an insufficient supply of blood. Treatment includes good blood sugar and blood pressure control, and the condition often improves on its own; sometimes, however, normal vision does not return. In some cases, intravitreal injections of steroids are helpful.

Retinal Vein Occlusion

As explained in the first chapter, retinal vein occlusion is a blockage of the veins that carry blood away from the retina. Individuals with diabetes have a higher than average risk of developing this blockage. This causes a condition similar to diabetic retinopathy in the eye with the blockage. The treatment is similar to that for diabetic retinopathy; this includes intravitreal anti-VEGF drugs, steroids, and focal laser photocoagulation for macular edema and panretinal laser photocoagulation if abnormal retinal vessels develop.

Corneal Erosion

The cornea is the layer of thin tissue on the surface of the eye. When this layer of tissue does not stay attached to the tissues below it, it creates a condition called *corneal erosion*. It is treated with lubricating eye ointments, particularly at bed-time. For acute episodes, eye patches may be used. Those with frequent recurrence of corneal erosion require specialized care by a general ophthalmologist or a corneal specialist.

In Summary

- Proliferative diabetic retinopathy require active treatments and should be monitored by regular evaluations.

- After diabetic macular edema or proliferative diabetic retinopathy develops, treatment with intravitreal injections or retinal laser photocoagulation is typically required.

- Individuals with diabetic macular edema may require regular evaluations and treatment until the condition is stabilized. Once stable, the interval between evaluations may become longer.

- Treatment of proliferative diabetic retinopathy includes panretinal laser photocoagulation (PRP). This may be performed in one or two sessions. The response to laser photocoagulation takes about two months to develop. Once the condition is stable, evaluation at regular intervals is recommended in order to detect and treat any recurrence at an early stage before too much damage is done.

- Some disorders caused by proliferative diabetic retinopathy may require a surgery, known as vitrectomy, which is the removal of the vitreous gel in the center of the eye.

- Although treatment for proliferative diabetic retinopathy can reduce further damage, it usually does not reverse the damage already done.

5 Reducing the Progression of Diabetic Retinopathy

When you have type 1 or type 2 diabetes, taking an active role in managing your disease is a critical part of maintaining eye health. Research consistently points to diabetes control as the most important factor in preventing irreversible damage to your vision.

Furthermore, there are other actions you can take to prevent complications of diabetes. Control other diseases such as high blood pressure and high cholesterol and lead a healthy life style. Eat a balanced diet, exercise, and control your weight. By doing so you can enjoy better overall health and preserve your vision.

Monitoring and Controlling Blood Sugar

Keeping your blood glucose as close to normal as possible is important in preventing or slowing the complications of diabetes, including diabetic retinopathy. Uncontrolled blood sugar accelerates damage to the small blood vessels in your retina, causing them to leak and become obstructed.

Your diabetes specialist will play a major role in advising you on nutrition and lifestyle changes. Your therapy plan begins with monitoring your blood sugar on a regular basis. You will need to test your blood sugar daily to make sure that it does not go too high or low. Ideally, that means a glucose level between 70 and 130 mg/dL before a meal and less than 180 mg/dL two hours after eating.

Another important test is the hemoglobin "A1c" blood test, which reflects a person's average blood glucose over the previous three months. The measure will tell your doctor how well your treatment is working. Check with your doctor about the right range for blood sugar and hemoglobin A1C for you.

If you need insulin—as all type 1 and many type 2 diabetics do—it is essential that you take it as prescribed by your physician. There are many aspects to controlling your diabetes and diabetic retinopathy. Monitoring and managing your blood glucose tops the list. Monitor your blood sugar, food intake, and time and dose of medication on a daily basis by keeping a record. Take these records with you when you visit with the physician who treats you for diabetes.

Research confirms that keeping blood glucose levels as close to normal as possible can slow the onset and progression of various diabetic-related complications, including diabetic retinopathy.

A major clinical study funded by the National Institute of Diabetes and Digestive and Kidney Diseases found that those with type 1 diabetes had the best health outcomes when they practiced intensive management of their diabetes. The study, called *The Diabetes Control and Complications Trial (DCCT)*, involved more than 1,400 type 1 diabetes participants who were evaluated over a decade. "Intensive management" meant study participants tried to keep hemoglobin A1C levels as close as possible to the normal value of 6 percent or less. Keeping blood glucose at this level slowed the onset and progression of eye disease as well as of kidney disease and nerve damage. These intensive practices include:

- testing blood glucose levels multiple times a day
- if needed, injecting insulin daily or using an insulin pump
- adjusting insulin dosages according to food intake and exercise
- following a diet and exercise plan
- seeing health care team members regularly

Intensive therapy not only reduced the risk of developing diabetic retinopathy by 76 percent, but also slowed the progression of eye damage by 54 percent in individuals with disease at the study's onset. Similar promising findings occurred for other diabetic complications, including 50 percent reduced risk for kidney disease and 60 percent reduced risk for nerve damage.

Although the *Epidemiology of Diabetes Interventions and Complications (EDIC) study* focused on patients with type 1 diabetes, the findings have similar implications for type 2 patients, since the blood vessels are harmed in comparable ways. *The United Kingdom Prospective Diabetes Study,* one of several clinical trials focusing specifically on type 2 diabetes, confirmed that good blood glucose control indeed leads to fewer diabetic complications, including eye disease.

Maintain Good Cardiovascular Health

Poor blood sugar control can also affect your cardiovasular health. The EDIC study showed intensive blood glucose control reduces the risk of any cardiovascular disease event by 42 percent and reduces the risk of heart attack, stroke, or death from cardiovascular causes by 57 percent.

Because cardiovascular diseases can increase the likelihood of diabetic complications, it is important that you control factors such as blood pressure and cholesterol levels. It also important to make routine exercise a part of your lifestyle; you should also quit smoking.

Control Blood Pressure

High blood pressure or "hypertension" is a condition in which the force of blood pushing against your artery walls rises above normal. Although the underlying cause for most cases of high blood pressure—referred to as "primary" or essential hypertension—is unknown, certain risk factors such as obesity, smoking, inactivity, a high-salt diet, and genetic factors play a role in its development and severity. As with diabetes, high blood pressure can affect your health in various ways.

Uncontrolled high blood pressure also plays a major role in the progression of diabetic retinopathy. Additionally, uncontrolled high blood pressure can make diabetic kidney damage worse.

According to both the American Diabetes Association (ADA) and the National Institutes of Health (NIH), most people with diabetes should aim for a blood pressure below 130/80 mmHg. Fortunately, there are effective ways to normalize your blood pressure.

Although treatment differs from person to person, the first course of action usually is to make simple lifestyle changes. Interventions such as maintaining a healthy weight and exercising regularly are important in controlling high blood pressure. Because salt intake influences blood pressure, your doctor also will recommend a low-salt diet. If lifestyle changes are not sufficient, your doctor may prescribe medication. Several types of drugs are effective in bringing blood pressure to a safe level.

Whatever the treatment, you need to have your blood pressure checked at regular intervals. Because blood pressure is an underlying factor in your retinopathy, it is important to monitor and manage it.

Control Cholesterol Levels

Contrary to what you might think, cholesterol is not entirely bad for your health. Normal levels of cholesterol found in your bloodstream and cells are necessary to help your body make vitamin D, hormones, and other important substances. Cholesterol levels outside normal ranges, however, are linked to heart and vascular diseases, including heart attack and stroke.

Unfortunately, diabetic individuals tend to have unhealthy cholesterol levels, which compounds the damage their disease is already doing to the blood vessels. Diabetes lowers good cholesterol, the *high-density lipoproteins* or *"HDLs"* that keep your vessels from narrowing with coronary artery disease–promoting plaque. Diabetes increases the bad cholesterol, the *low-density lipoproteins* or *"LDLs"* that facilitate blockage of blood vessels. It also raises *triglycerides,* another important form of fat in the body. In excess, triglycerides contribute significantly to the *atherosclerotic* plaque or hardening of the arteries in the heart and other vital organs.

As a person with diabetes, you need to manage your cholesterol tightly, not just for your cardiovascular system, but also for the benefits it will provide for other organs that rely on healthy blood vessels such as the eye, the kidney, and the brain. Because studies have shown that increased blood lipids are associated with macular edema, controlling these can help reduce further damage to your eyesight. Your doctor will discuss your target blood lipid level. For individuals with diabetes, the American Diabetes Association recommends an annual blood test to monitor cholesterol and triglyceride levels. Normal blood lipid levels are:

- LDL cholesterol: less than 100 mg/dL
- HDL cholesterol: above 40 mg/dL for men and above 50 mg/dL for women
- Triglycerides: less than 150 mg/dL

The good news about improving your cholesterol is that the same lifestyle changes that work to lower your blood pressure—losing weight; exercising more;

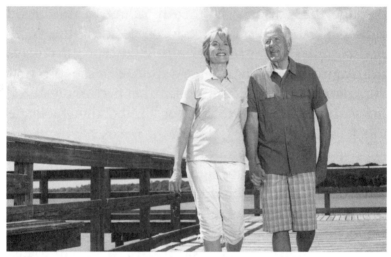

Regular exercise is an important part of controlling blood sugar levels. Exercise increases circulation and helps the body use insulin more efficiently.

adopting a low-fat, high fiber diet; and abstaining from tobacco—will yield blood cholesterol benefits, too. If lifestyle modifications are not enough, your physician may prescribe medication to control lipid levels. Fortunately, the medications can be very effective.

Exercise Regularly

Physical activity is another important factor in controlling diabetes, high blood pressure, high cholesterol, and their associated complications, such as diabetic retinopathy. Research consistently points to the role of aerobic exercise and strength building in lowering blood sugar and helping the body use insulin efficiently. It can also reduce weight while decreasing blood pressure and blood cholesterol, three key risk factors in both diabetes and cardiovascular disease.

Unless you hear differently from your physician, any activity that ups your heart rate or helps build muscle mass is a positive step. You do not have to join a gym or run a marathon to experience the health benefits. Walking briskly, swimming, bicycling, or playing tennis thirty minutes a day, three to five days a week, will help with your insulin response and improve your circulation. By lifting weights and doing resistance exercises two to three times a week, you can also build muscle mass. The more muscle you have, the more efficient your body will be at burning calories and regulating your blood sugar. Whatever exercise plan your doctor thinks will work for you, physical activity can benefit every part of your body, including your eyes.

Quit Smoking

Tobacco can do great harm to your blood vessels even if you don't have diabetes. It increases the process of atherosclerosis, intensifying hardening of the arteries caused by other factors. When your vessels are already compromised by diabetes, smoking compounds the problem by increasing their susceptibility to damage. Research also shows that smoking can cause oxidative damage in the macula as well as interfere with the absorption of *lutein,* a micronutrient that protects the retinal cells.

Quitting smoking can be a challenge. Tobacco is an addiction that is difficult to break. But when you have diabetic retinopathy, you have motivation beyond just shielding your coronary vessels. Abstaining from smoking can help you protect your retinal vessels, too. Fortunately, there are many methods to help you successfully quit: nicotine patches, gum, sprays, counseling, behavior modification, and even hypnosis.

There are also medications that might be helpful, including the drug Chantix *(varenicline)*. Chantix stimulates nicotine receptors more weakly than nicotine itself, therefore reducing the need for nicotine. It both reduces cravings for and decreases the pleasurable effects of cigarettes and other tobacco products. Through these mechanisms, it can help some patients give up smoking. You may have to make many attempts before you are successful at giving up smoking, but the benefits to your overall health will be well worth the effort.

Practice Good Nutrition

A balanced, nutritious diet will help improve your overall health as well as control your diabetes. A diet low in fat, cholesterol, salt, and added sugar but high in certain fruits, vegetables, complex carbohydrates, and fiber (whole-grain breads and cereals, and oat bran) is important in controlling your blood sugar, as well as reducing your weight, blood pressure, and cholesterol. Making food choices that lower these risk factors will protect your eyesight as well as your heart.

Eat Fruits and Vegetables

Research has shown that certain micronutrients such as *vitamin E, vitamin C, zinc, copper, lutein,* and *zeaxanthin* offer specific protection against another serious eye disease, macular degeneration. With diabetic retinopathy, the antioxidant effects are more general in nature. Fruits and leafy green vegetables are a great source of these vitamins, minerals, and phytochemicals your body needs to function well. Because they are fiber-filled and often low in calories, fruits and vegetables can help you reach and maintain a healthy weight.

Choosing Fats Wisely

In terms of a healthy diet, fat sometimes gets a bad reputation. Every meal plan designed to reduce weight and decrease blood cholesterol, blood pressure, and glucose suggests low-fat foods. But not all fats are equal. Yes, you need to avoid the "bad" fats because they can be harmful to your overall health, especially if you have diabetes. The "bad" fats include:

- *saturated fats:* found primarily in animal products such as meat and dairy, they raise LDLs or bad cholesterol levels.

- *trans fats:* found in processed foods such as store-bought chips, cookies, and crackers, they can raise LDLs and lower HDLs or the good fats.

But you need to include the "good" fats that promote health, such as:

- *monosaturated fats:* found in a variety of oils and foods such as olive oil and avocados, these fats promote healthy cholesterol levels while decreasing the risk of cardiovascular disease.

- *polyunsaturated fats:* found in plant-based foods and oils, these fats improve cholesterol levels. Omega-3 fatty acids, which have known cardiovascular benefits, are readily available in many food products:
  - salmon and other cold-water fish such as herring and tuna
  - flaxseed and flaxseed oil
  - walnuts and walnut oil
  - other oils such as olive, grapeseed, and canola

Eating the right fats can have a positive impact on your cardiovascular health, which benefits your diabetes and ultimately your diabetic retinopathy.

Choosing Carbohydrates

Because complex carbohydrates are the most important energy source for your body, you need to include them in your diet. But there are differences in carbohydrates based on their chemical structure. "Simple" carbohydrates are those found in processed and refined foods that contain white flour and sugar. These include pastries and candies, as well as certain fruits and milk products. Even if the food does not contain sugar, the simple carbohydrates themselves quickly turn into sugar after you eat them.

Limit your intake of these foods because they cause rapid spikes in your blood sugar levels and also contribute to weight gain. Make sure your diet includes "complex" carbohydrates—the starches and fiber found in whole-grain breads and cereals, dried beans, lentils, and peas. The combination of fiber and

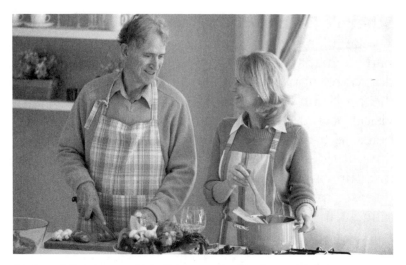

A balanced diet plays a crucial role in managing blood sugar levels.

natural sugars in these foods digests more slowly than simple sugars and does not create the spikes in blood sugar levels. Fiber is also known to lower blood pressure and control cholesterol; it also makes you feel full longer, which can be helpful in losing weight. For those reasons, being selective in, and balancing your dietary carbohydrates, can help you manage your diabetes, which benefits your eyes.

Have a meal plan and follow it routinely. A dietitian can work with you to develop a meal plan by including foods that you and your family like to eat and that are good for you, too. Keep a record of the type and amount of food that you eat so you can monitor and, if necessary, modify your diet to achieve better diabetes control.

Schedule Regular Eye Examinations

Regular eye examinations are a very important part of managing diabetic retinopathy. Early detection of retinopathy allows your eye specialist to treat the problem before irreversible damage and loss of vision occurs. Although diabetic retinopathy, like diabetes, is a chronic condition that can progress over time, it does not need to cause irreversible damage to your vision. By monitoring and controlling your disease, making healthy lifestyle choices, and being diligent in your eye evaluations, you can lower the risk of losing your sight.

In Summary

- You can reduce the progression of diabetic retinopathy and risk of vision loss by making these steps a part of your lifestyle:
  - regular eye examinations
  - treatment of diabetic retinopathy complications before severe damage occurs
  - tight control of diabetes
  - good blood pressure control
  - good blood lipid control
  - healthful diet
  - physical activity
  - weight control
  - abstinence from smoking
- Taken together, these actions can have a positive impact on your diabetes, as well as on your cardiovascular system, kidneys, and general health.

- Regular visits to your diabetes and primary care physician, following your doctors' instructions, compliance with any medication that is prescribed, and making healthy lifestyle choices are all important factors for minimizing vision damage and other complications of diabetes.

6 Coping with Vision Impairment

If your diabetic retinopathy has caused vision loss, you will need to make adjustments. Fortunately, you do not have to go it alone. Resources are available in most communities to help visually challenged individuals deal with many aspects of their lives. Your eye specialist can refer you to professionals, experts in the techniques and tools necessary to accommodate your diminished sight. The strategies they suggest not only will help you administer your diabetes medication more safely, but may also help you to meet many other visual challenges. Mastering them can make the activities of daily living much easier.

Professionals Who Can Help

If you are experiencing bothersome vision loss due to diabetic retinopathy, your eye specialist will refer you to experts who can assist you in adjusting. Fortunately, many of these professionals are not only expert in helping people with limited or reduced vision, but also familiar with the special challenges of diabetic retinopathy.

Diabetes Educators

If you have been diagnosed with diabetes, you may already be working with a *certified diabetes educator*. These are health care professionals—nurses, dietitians, pharmacists, exercise physiologists, podiatrists, and others—whose job is to aid individuals in understanding and managing their disease. A diabetes educator will help you find a glucose meter and insulin delivery system that not only meets your medical needs but also accommodates your vision challenges. Likewise, he or she can teach you safe and effective techniques for self-testing and treatment that do not require perfect sight.

Low-Vision Specialists

These professionals are usually licensed doctors of optometry who have undergone specialized training in prescribing low-vision lenses and devices. They are very familiar with ways of enhancing all aspects of daily living. Because diabetes, specifically diabetic retinopathy, is a leading cause of blindness, low-vision specialists are very familiar with the self-management goals linked to this disease. They can also help you with devices and techniques for measuring your glucose and administering insulin.

A low-vision expert also can help you weigh the pros and cons—cost, effectiveness, and the "ergonomics" or ease of use—of many vision devices. He or she will take into account your work, lifestyle, environment, and routine in matching resources to your needs. If a professional suggests a home visit to make your house "eye friendly," rest assured that such a visit could be very beneficial.

Also, remember that adjusting to any low-vision device, whether directly related to your diabetes or otherwise, is not immediate. It will take time and effort to use the new tools in your life effectively. If you have progressive retinopathy, you may find that the strategies and devices you have selected may become ineffective as your condition worsens. You will need to work with your low-vision specialist to accommodate the changes, even if that means refining your nonvisual skills.

Low-Vision Aids

Although navigating all aspects of your life can be challenging if you are visually impaired from diabetic retinopathy, testing your glucose daily and administering insulin are likely the most pressing tasks. Fortunately, with devices available today you can perform many tasks with relative ease; for example you can purchase glucose meters that "talk" and you tell you your glucose levels and prefilled insulin syringes that resemble ballpoint pens. The key is in working with your diabetes educator and low-vision specialist to find the right combination.

"Talking" Meters

If you have moderate to severe vision loss, you will likely need more than a traditional blood glucose monitor, even if it has enlarged digital numbers and backlighting. Fortunately, advances in technology have made talking glucose meters—monitors that emit instructions and deliver results aloud—readily available and relatively inexpensive.

Of the two types of audio monitors, the first type combines an off-the-shelf glucose meter with external voice hardware to convert displayed text into audible speech. The second type has a built-in audio function. Beyond those major differences, there are other features that can be found in various models. Some meters speak in both English and Spanish. That includes guiding you through each blood-testing step, advising if you have made an error, or warning you that your battery is low. You may also be able to confirm your results or retrieve past scores from the meter's memory.

Because there are many glucose meters on the market, it is important to work with a diabetes educator or low-vision expert to identify the best unit for you. He or she can help you weigh the various features, especially as they apply to your diminished vision. You will likely have many questions to ask about your options, but the ones specific to talking models might include:

- Does this meter have a built-in voice function? If not, can I add a voice attachment?
- Does the unit speak in a language other than English? Is it easy to understand?
- Will the meter talk me through the setup or do I need sighted help?
- Will the meter guide me through steps of blood glucose testing or just give me spoken results?

- Does this meter also have tactile markings on the surface to help me place a test strip in the right place?
- Can I retrieve past results from memory and will they be spoken?

Beyond the audio function, you will also need to know if the test strips for a particular model are relatively simple to insert and use. Do you have to code the meter with every new box? Can you insert a strip easily despite your vision limitations? How do you ensure that a drop of blood hits the strip correctly if you cannot see it well? Someone familiar with the latest products, especially the newest palm-sized units, can help you identify a technique for inserting the strip, lancing your finger, and making sure that your blood drop hits the mark.

If your vision is poor now, it may be a factor in selecting a glucose meter. Even though many of the newer monitors are equipped with speech chips or add-on voice synthesizers, you may still have to rely on your tactile senses or vision for some functions. You may find it helpful to put a large permanent mark on the unit where the strip needs to be inserted as well as work with colored lancing devices.

Whether they "talk" or not, today's glucose meters are smaller and simpler to use and require smaller blood samples than models of the past. They also offer a variety of features, such as memory storage and computer connections, that allow you to view your blood sugar results on an even bigger screen.

Insulin Pens

Measuring insulin accurately can be a challenge, especially if you have partial or complete vision loss. Fortunately, many insulin delivery system designs are available to help visually impaired individuals.

Although the conventional way to get insulin into your body is with vial and syringe, an *insulin pen* can ease the injection process. They come in two basic models, both of which are relatively simple to use in terms of loading medication and delivering the injection. Disposable pens are prefilled whereas reusable models deliver insulin via inserted cartridges. In terms of getting the correct dosage, you either count the number of audible clicks as the units appear on an electronic display or feel the raised spots on a mechanical kitchen-timer-like dial, until you reach the right number of units.

With any insulin pen, you will still have to insert a micro-fine needle for each injection. A diabetes educator or low-vision specialist can help you navigate the steps. Even though insulin pens are generally easier to operate than conventional vial-and-syringe methods, they can be dangerous if used improperly. As such, many pens carry manufacturer warnings against low-vision or blind individuals using the device independently. An expert can help you determine if using the device is a safe option for you.

Insulin Pumps

Some individuals with diabetes find that an insulin pump, a computerized palm-sized device that you wear around your waist, is the best match to their life-

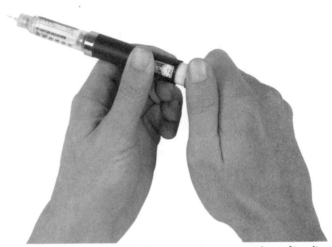

An insulin injection pen resembles a ballpoint pen. It uses cartridges of insulin and disposable needles.

style. Instead of periodic injections through the day, the pump delivers rapid-acting insulin continuously via a *catheter*. More specifically, insulin passes from a reservoir inside the pump into the body via a thin tube. It connects to a *cannula* or a tiny reedlike needle permanently inserted under the skin. The pump is programmed to deliver correct dosages, which are released in two ways: a *basal,* or continuous level, between meals, during exercise, or at night; or a *bolus,* or instant larger dosage, just before meals. There are numerous advantages to an insulin pump, not the least of which is that diabetes management is easier and more accurate because of the programmed dosages. But there are disadvantages. It can be bothersome to be attached to the pump most of the time. You also need to be trained to use it. Your diabetes educator can help you weigh the pros and cons in determining if a pump is right for you.

Prefilled Syringes

Having a sighted person fill a number of syringes for you is a very doable option if you are still administering the medication via the traditional vial-and-syringe method. Filled syringes can be kept in the refrigerator for up to thirty days. Some pharmacies even offer this service. If you prefill syringes yourself, make sure you store them pointing upwards so they do not become clogged with suspended insulin particles. If you store a number of premixed syringes, or syringes that contain two different types of insulin, make sure to roll the syringe between your hands to mix the solutions prior to injection.

Other Insulin Delivery Devices

If you still inject your insulin using syringe and vial, there are ways to ensure that you draw the correct amount, especially if you are visually impaired. Magnifying guides that fit over the syringe, for instance, not only enlarge the measures, but also hold the insulin bottle firmly in place while you draw the correct dosage. Some models can also aid in inserting the needle and even locating bubbles in the syringe. Magnifiers are inexpensive and readily available through pharmacies and online suppliers.

You may benefit from a variety of other devices on the market to help visually impaired diabetics measure insulin dosages, draw the medication into the syringe, and guide the needle through injection, including:

- dosage counting devices that enable users to draw and mix correct doses of up to two insulin types. With each unit drawn into the syringe, these devices emit a distinct click that can be heard and felt so no vision is required.

- caps or other fittings that guide the syringe needle as it's inserted into an insulin bottle
- syringe "loaders" that can be adjusted to ensure the same exact insulin amounts dose after dose
- syringes with colored plungers that make reading calibration numbers easier
- devices placed on the skin to guide the needle during injection

Some insulin delivery systems and aids work best for people with partial sight and others work well if you are nearly or completely blind. A professional familiar with the alternatives can advise you as to what devices will match your insulin requirements and visual needs.

Other Low-Vision Aids

Whether you need to monitor or treat your diabetes or just perform the tasks of daily living, there are many specially designed gadgets available to help you navigate with visual impairment. Many of the following items are available either at office supply stores or online:

- magnifiers
- telescopic devices
- video magnifiers
- reading machines

- eyeglass filters
- voice-activated note takers
- record-keeping and check-writing aids
- computers
- phones, clocks, and other devices

Magnifiers

Special magnifying devices are relatively inexpensive and efficient tools for taking on "close-up" or "near" vision. That includes doing detailed work or reading small print of any sort, especially unit markings on insulin syringes and glucose meter displays. Magnifiers come in various forms to suit your needs and preferences. Strength ranges from two to twenty times the actual size, depending on the model.

Handheld magnifiers. Known commonly as magnifying glasses, these handy little tools come in a range of dimensions and magnification power up to five times the actual size. You can adjust the clarity quickly by simply varying the distance between your eyes and the objects to be viewed. Some models are equipped with battery-operated lighting, casting additional illumination on hard-to-read material. The disadvantages of handheld magnifiers are that they offer a limited visual field and relatively low magnification in comparison to other tools. They also are difficult to use if your hands shake. Nevertheless, they are low cost and portable. You can take them almost anywhere.

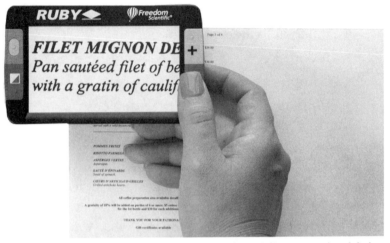

Handheld video magnifiers can be used for reading small print, product labels, medicine bottle labels, menus, or appliance controls.
Photo courtesy of Freedom Scientific.

Stand magnifiers. Larger than handheld magnifiers, stand magnifiers come in many different styles, all of which can aid you in reading, writing, and other detailed tasks. They are either mounted on stands placed directly on a flat surface or attached to desk or floor lamps. In fact, stand magnifiers commonly come with a light source. Like lamps used by a dentist or watch repairer, magnifying lamps illuminate and enlarge a specific area. Although they resemble ordinary adjustable-arm desk or floor lamps, the light source surrounds the lens in either a rectangle or circle. You simply position the magnifier over material for a close-up view. The disadvantages of stand magnifiers include higher cost and lack of portability. The advantages are higher magnification and steadiness.

Telescopic Devices

Besides facilitating "near" vision, you will likely need help with distance viewing as well. Fortunately, there are many devices available today to help you do both. Binoculars, monoculars, and enhanced eyeglasses are equipped telescopically to enlarge figures at a distance or microscopically for close-ups.

Binocular/monocular telescopes. The "bi" in binoculars refers to both eyes. These specialized low-vision telescopic devices help in focusing on distant objects. They are useful for watching television and viewing sporting and other big-venue events. (Some models are also designed for magnification of close-up tasks.) Most binoculars allow you to adjust each eye separately for maximum clarity. The "mono" in *monoculars* refers to one eye only. Monoculars are helpful for many of the same reasons as binoculars. They are also small, portable, inexpensive, and available in a range of magnification powers.

Eyeglass-mounted devices. Small telescopes can be attached to a pair of eyeglasses to enhance distance vision. Usually available by prescription, telescopic devices can be monocular or binocular.

They are either clipped temporarily to the frames or mounted permanently on the lens. They also may be attached to the upper part of your glasses so you have use of the bottom half for closer tasks. They free your hands and facilitate doing things at "arm's length," such as reading the computer screen where you have downloaded your glucose test results.

Because both magnifiers and telescopes each have their own advantages and disadvantages, you

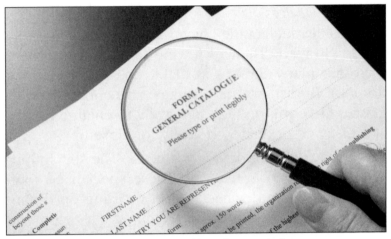

Handheld magnifying glasses are portable and economical.

may want to try several devices or even switch from one to another, depending on the task. A low-vision specialist can help you evaluate your needs plus the trade-offs among different options because they differ in terms of magnification levels, working distances, and field-of-view. A common rule of thumb is the stronger the magnification, the smaller the field of vision and the closer the device has to be to your eye.

Keep in mind that walking while looking through any magnifying device can be hazardous because your side vision, depth perception, and balance will be affected.

Video Magnifiers

Also known as *closed-circuit televisions (CCTVs),* video magnifiers use a stand-mounted or handheld camera to capture an image placed beneath it. It's enlarged and projected on a video monitor, television, or computer screen. The downsides of video magnifiers are the relatively high cost and the reduced field of vision. The upsides are that they can magnify anything, including medicine labels and instructions, placed under the camera. A stand-mounted video also frees you to test your blood glucose or fill an insulin syringe with magnification.

Reading Machines

Available in desktop or portable models, reading machines scan handwritten or printed material and then recite it back aloud. Because the device can convert any text to speech, you can read books, newspapers, magazines, food labels, prescriptions, and many more items. Any computer can become a reading machine with the addition of a specialized program called *optical character recognition* software.

Eyeglass Filters

Specialized colored clear acetate or plastic sheets, called *absorptive filters,* can help you get the most from your vision while reading. They increase contrasts, reduce glare, and ease the transition between light backgrounds and dark figures. These filters are available in a variety of colors, including yellow, amber, or marigold.

Voice-Activated Note Takers

Reminding yourself to check your glucose and take your insulin can be simple and easy with a voice-activated note taker. Many handheld digital recorders offer this feature, which can be readily adapted for

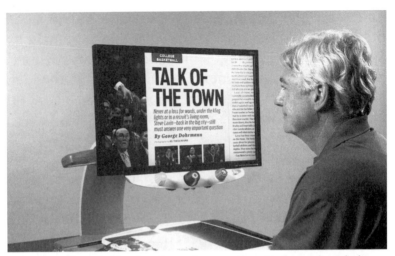

Video magnifiers provide crisp, clear enlargements and help you do such things as read small print, sign checks, or write letters. *Photo courtesy of Freedom Scientific.*

creating to-do or shopping lists and even taking notes at meetings. Because the devices are small, they fit easily in a pocket or purse.

Record-Keeping and Check-Writing Aids

If you are visually impaired, you do not have to give up your financial independence. A number of low-vision aids can help you write your own checks and perform other record-keeping tasks. Signature guides, for instance, will help you place your name appropriately on checks, contracts, and other documents. You can also order checks with raised lettering or large print from many banks.

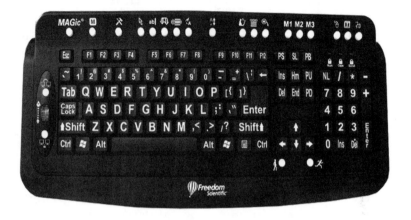

Large-print keyboards make it easier to work at a computer.
Photo courtesy of Freedom Scientific.

Computers

There are a number of helpful products on the market today designed for low-vision individuals. Computers can be modified, for instance, with large-print, high contrast keyboards that are easier to see even in low light. They can be outfitted with larger monitors and screen magnifiers that enlarge images. You can also install both voice recognition programs that allow you to verbally command the computer and screen-reading software that translates text into spoken words.

Phones, Clocks, and Other Numbered Devices

Technology is helping visually impaired individuals in other ways. Phones are now available with larger, lighted numbers, making it easier to place and receive calls. Some have voice functions so you can speak the commands. In addition to larger digital numbers, clocks, wristwatches, and timers of all types often can tell time either by speech or vibration. Calculators are readily available with large-number, high-contrast buttons and high-contrast displays for enhanced visibility.

Coping with Decreasing Vision in Your Home

Incorporating simple strategies in your daily routine can help you adapt to vision changes due to diabetic retinopathy. By making changes in your physical surroundings, organizing what is around you, and relying increasingly on your other senses, you can navigate the day with confidence and ease.

Improve Lighting

Because insufficient illumination and glare can be a problem with diabetic retinopathy, you should have your surroundings evaluated for lighting. Many low-vision experts make house visits to analyze the environment and suggest changes. The good news is that you can make significant improvements with simple measures such as positioning floor lamps, desk lamps, and magnifying lights strategically; improving lighting in entryways, stairways, and basements; and using dimmer switches, night lights, and motion-activated light sensors to vary lighting levels to prevent accidents in the dark.

You will want to target where you work, read, and perform detailed tasks such as testing your glucose or filling a syringe. A flexible-arm lamp, for instance, that can be adjusted to a variety of tasks and settings provides critical lighting for close vision.

Get Organized

Many individuals who are visually impaired find it very helpful to get and stay organized. Establishing consistency and routine in all things can greatly reduce your frustrations. To prevent trips and falls, for instance, eliminate clutter around your house. To prevent important documents from getting lost, place bills, keys, reading material, and other items into clearly labeled bins or baskets. Also, keeping everything in a designated place on your countertops and in drawers and cupboards simplifies everyday tasks such as preparing food, bathing, and getting dressed.

Sharpen Your Other Senses

If your vision becomes significantly impaired because of diabetic retinopathy, you will need to rely increasingly on your other senses. Learning to use touch and hearing effectively can help you adjust to an environment you no longer can see clearly. Marking different insulin bottles with rubber bands or textured tape, for instance, can help you identify the correct vial if colored tape, stickers, and felt-tip pens no longer work. The same techniques work for separating other items that you use in your daily life.

Sharpening your listening skills can be very beneficial. You can use glucose meters and insulin delivery systems that alert you via synthesized speech or audio cues. Similarly, many magazines, newspapers, and books are available on tape so "reading" requires good listening skills.

Coping in Your Workplace

Being able to function outside your living environment is a large part of being independent. It is important to craft a coping strategy for the workplace so you feel comfortable and are able to work productively. A critical first step may be to speak with your employer about your limitations and any accommodations that might help you. In addition to suggesting possible changes in your workspace, bring whatever strategies—improved lighting, organization and routine, and reliance on your other senses—that have worked at home to your office and work activities. They likely will enhance your productivity.

Enjoying Travel and Recreation

Just because you have diabetic retinopathy doesn't mean you can't explore the world or otherwise enjoy your leisure time. Each year, millions of visually impaired individuals travel successfully and participate in recreational activities, despite their eyesight limitations. Just like them, you can benefit from advanced planning, specialized tools, and other assistance widely available in many leisure-related industries.

Travel

Whether you want to take off to exotic places or just explore closer to home, you will find many services that can help you achieve your goals. Travel agencies often specialize in booking trips for people with specific disabilities, including low vision. Directories of such agencies are available online. In addition, many airlines, cruise lines, train stations, and hotels offer assistance, even discounts, for visually impaired individuals. Check their websites for more information. When traveling, keep these tips in mind:

- Always arrive early at the airport, train station, bus station, or cruise ship port to allow enough time for navigating the area.

- Notify customer service representatives that you are visually impaired and need additional help to your departure gate or baggage claim area.

- Preboard so you have plenty of time to find your seat and stow your carry-on baggage.

- Use bright, colorful tags to identify your luggage or use brightly colored bags.

- Whenever possible, rent the audio tour of a tourist attraction. It may even be free if you have visual limitations.

Recreation

Even with vision impairment, you can still enjoy many different games, hobbies, and other recreational activities. Thanks to today's visual aids, you can carry on with activities you love, despite visual limitations.

Games/hobbies. Board games and playing cards are widely available in large-print editions, as are books of popular word games and puzzles. A growing number of video games that use sound cues instead of images are available for the visually impaired.

Gardening. If you love gardening, you need not let reduced vision prevent you from pursuing it. There are things you can do to make this a safer hobby: Create a walkway through your garden using non-slippery surfaces so you don't trip; choose gardening tools with brightly colored handles; and select plants in bright colors so you can enjoy them.

Exercising. Because physical activity is paramount in controlling your diabetes, you want to do everything possible to exercise routinely. A stationary bike or treadmill is an ideal at-home aerobic option. Other forms of exercise that you can do with visual limitations include weight training for muscle strengthening and yoga for balance, flexibility, and focus. With the right training, and safety techniques, you can even swim. Exercise is good for every part of your body.

Staying Connected Socially

As a visually impaired person you may find it challenging to keep in touch with and communicate your needs to others. But having a social network and adapting to social situations is critical for your emotional health. By being part of a larger community, you not only expand your circle of friends, but also meet those who might help you when you need help. The key is to be open about your visual limitations and be willing to ask for assistance.

Friends and family. Engaging those closest to you in your coping strategies is important. It is important to let family and friends know how they can assist you, even if the request is as simple as asking people to put things back in their original place. As you go through the day, you may encounter friends, family members, and even strangers who want to help you by opening a door, finding an elevator button, or even helping you up the steps. Depending on your vision loss, you may simply want to thank them for their offer but indicate that you are doing fine. If you need help, however, do not hesitate to ask for it.

Social situations. Whatever your vision loss, you will likely need to adapt to social situations. Although it is common in our society to look someone in the eye when meeting or saying hello, if diabetic retinopathy has involved your macula or central vision, you may have difficulty doing so. In fact, you may have to move your eyes up, down, or to the side to use your peripheral vision in finding another person's facial features. It is a good idea to let people know that you have a vision problem so they understand why you cannot look them straight in the eye. It may even be a conversation starter.

Finding outside support. As a visually impaired person you want to be as independent as possible. But you do not want that independence to lead to isolation. Joining a support group can have many positive effects on your life. It can help you emotionally while putting you in touch with others facing the same challenges. A group setting offers an opportunity to share your thoughts openly and even swap strategies on coping with daily life.

Scheduling Regular Retinal Evaluations

Whatever the stage of your diabetic retinopathy, regular comprehensive eye evaluations and treatments will be an important part of your life. A dilated eye examination may seem time consuming and inconvenient, but it is critical in saving your remaining sight. Keep in mind that even if you have severe proliferative retinopathy, you can still have 20/20 or normal vision and no outward signs of the disease. So just checking your eyes for a corrective lens prescription is not enough. The only way your doctor can know if your vision is threatened is to evaluate your macula and peripheral retina routinely. Once your condition is diagnosed and treated, you need to follow-up with regular examinations. Because diabetic retinopathy is an ongoing problem, you will have to pay attention to it your entire life.

But, however severe your vision loss from diabetic retinopathy is, you can learn to adapt to most daily activities with the help of technology, friends and family, and medical supervision.

In Summary

A diabetes educator or low-vision specialist can refer you to products and techniques that can enhance your life.

- There are many tools to help you monitor and control your diabetes if you have low vision.

- An array of specialized devices will help you navigate other parts of your life despite your vision impairment.

- By adopting various coping strategies at home, in your workplace, and while traveling or engaging in leisure activities, you do not have to let your visual limitations prevent you from enjoying a full and productive lifestyle.

- Friends, family, and support groups can have a positive, helpful effect on your life.

Resources

American Academy of Ophthalmology
P.O. Box 7424
San Francisco, CA 94120-7424
Phone: (415) 561-8500
www.aao.org

American Association of Diabetes Educators
200 W. Madison Street, Suite 800
Chicago, IL 60606
Phone: (800) 338-3633
www.diabeteseducator.org

American Diabetes Association
1701 North Beauregard Street
Alexandria, VA 22311
Phone: (800) 342-2383
www.diabetes.org

American Foundation for the Blind
2 Penn Plaza, Suite 1102
New York, NY 10121
Phone: (212) 502-7600
www.afb.org

American Optometric Association
243 North Lindbergh Boulevard
St. Louis, MO 63141
Phone: (800) 365-2219
www.aoa.org

American Society of Retina Specialists
20 North Wacker Drive, Suite 2234
Chicago, IL 60606
Phone: (312) 578-8760
www.asrs.org

Association for Macular Diseases, Inc.
210 East 64th Street
New York, NY 10065
Phone: (212) 605-3719
www.macula.org

National Diabetes Information Clearing House
1 Information Way
Bethesda, MD 20892-3560
Phone: (800) 860-8747
www.diabetes.niddk.nih.gov

National Eye Institute/
National Institutes of Health
2020 Vision Place
Bethesda, MD 20892-3655
Phone: (301) 496-5248
www.nei.nih.gov

National Federation of the Blind
200 East Wells Street at Jernigan Place
Baltimore, MD 21230
Phone: (410) 659-9314
www.nfb.org

Retina Vitreous Associates
9001 Wilshire Boulavard., Suite. 301
Beverly Hills, CA 90211
Phone: (310) 854-6201
www.laretina.com
www.maculainfo.org
www.retinainfo.org

Glossary

A

Age-related macular degeneration (AMD): A degenerative condition that affects the center portion of the retina known as the macula. AMD is the leading cause of legal blindness in individuals over the age of fifty years.

Amsler grid: A grid with a dot in the center, used to test for symptoms that may signify macular disease.

Angiography: The process of obtaining images of blood vessels within and under the retina that retina specialists use to diagnose many of the retinal diseases. *See also* Fundus fluorecein angiography.

Anterior chamber: Fluid-filled space inside the eye behind the cornea and in front of the iris.

Antioxidant: An agent that reduces the damage due to by-products of the normal chemical reactions with oxygen in the body.

Anti-VEGF drugs: Anti-vascular endothelial growth factor drugs that target abnormal blood vessel growth and leakage.

Arteriosclerosis: Thickening and hardening of the walls of the arteries.

Artery: Blood vessel that carries oxygenated blood to the tissues of the body.

Atherosclerosis: The accumulation of fatty deposits on the walls of large blood vessels.

B

Beta-carotene: A type of vitamin A.

Blind spots: A commonly reported symptom of macular disease in which patients report that areas of their vision are missing.

Blood pressure: Pressure exerted on the walls of vessels by circulation of blood. Measurements are indicated as "systolic," for pressure as the heart contracts (the "top" number), and "diastolic," for pressure when the heart is at rest (the "bottom" number).

Blurring: A commonly reported symptom of eye disease in which patients report that lines or edges of objects lose their sharpness.

Body Mass Index (BMI): Calculated from a person's height versus weight, body mass index indicates your body fat. It is often cited as a risk for certain health conditions, including diabetes and heart disease.

Bruch's membrane: A thin, compact layer of fibers located between the retinal pigment epithelium (RPE) of the retina and the underlying flat carpet of blood vessels and choroid that supplies the retina with nourishment.

B-scan ultrasonography: Use of high-frequency sound waves to reveal cross-sectional two-dimensional images of the inner eye. This technique is used when direct visualization of retina is not possible.

C

Capillaries: The smallest blood vessels in the body. Capillaries form a meshwork of small blood vessels that transport the blood from the arteries, through the body tissues, to the veins.

Carbohydrates: As one of the most important sources of energy for the body, these nutrients are converted into glucose through digestion. Carbohydrates are labeled as "simple" or "complex" depending on their chemical structure. Simple carbohydrates are found in fruits, vegetables, milk, and milk products as well as the sugars added during food processing and refining. Complex carbohydrates include whole grain breads and cereals, starchy vegetables, and legumes, many of which are good sources of fiber. For a healthy diet, limit the amount of added sugar and choose whole grains over refined grains.

Cataract: A clouding of the lens that causes decreased vision. People with diabetic retinopathy are at increased risk for age-related cataracts (called *nuclear sclerotic cataracts*). A special type of cataract, posterior subcapsular cataract, is most commonly seen in diabetic individuals.

Catheter: Flexible tubing inserted into a cavity of the body to introduce or withdraw fluid.

CCTV (Closed-circuit television): A technology that uses a video camera to project objects on a screen at increased magnification by simply placing them under the camera.

Central vision: Vision used for reading and fine detail work.

Certified diabetes educator: Professional trained to assist newly diagnosed diabetics with monitoring, treating, and living with diabetes.

Cholesterol: A type of lipid (fat) that can accumulate on the walls of arteries and cause health problems. The body produces all the cholesterol it needs without adding any to the diet.

Choroid: A specialized tissue layer that contains a network of blood vessels and is located under the retina.

Choroidal neovascularization (CNV): A process in which abnormal blood vessels grow from the small blood vessels in the choroid under the retina. This is the hallmark of wet macular degeneration.

Conjunctiva: A mucus membrane that lines the inside of the eyelids and extends over the front of the white part of the eye. This is the thin, loose layer of tissue that covers the eye.

Cornea: The transparent front part of the eye that helps focus the image. It is often referred to as the "window" of the eye.

D

Diabetes mellitus *(MEL-ih-tus)*: Group of diseases characterized by high blood glucose or sugar levels resulting from the body's inability to produce and/or use insulin. *Type 1 diabetes* occurs when the body produces little or no insulin. *Type 2 diabetes* occurs when the body does not produce enough insulin or the cells ignore it. "Gestational" diabetes appears only during pregnancy and normally disappears after delivery.

Diabetic retinopathy: Damage to the retina, the light-sensitive tissue at the back of the eye, because of uncontrolled blood glucose. It causes the tiny vessels of the retina to leak blood and fluid, ultimately interfering with vision. The two major types include: nonproliferative diabetic retinopathy (NPDR), characterized by damage to normal vessels, and proliferative diabetic retinopathy (PDR), characterized by abnormal new vessel growth.

Diagnose: To determine the cause of an illness or medical condition.

Dilate: To enlarge the pupils.

Disability: An impairment that affects one's ability to perform certain daily functions.

Distortion of vision: A commonly reported symptom of macular disease in which patients report that straight lines appear wavy.

E

Epiretinal membrane: Thin sheet of fibrous material that develop abnormally on the surface of the macula, causing wrinkling of the macula, visual blurring, and distortion.

F

Floaters: These are particles that float in the vitreous and create shadows on the retina. Floaters may take any shape and size; usually they are in the form of dots, curved lines, or a net.

Fluorescein: A special dye used for visualizing blood vessels of the retina and choroid.

Fovea: The center part of the macula that provides the sharpest vision.

Free radicals: Toxic substances produced by all cells.

Fundus fluorescein angiography (FA): Technique used for visualizing blood vessels in the retina and choroid. *See also* Angiography.

G

Glaucoma: Disorder of the eye characterized by an increase

120

of pressure within the eyeball. "Neovascular glaucoma" occurs during diabetic retinopathy when abnormal new vessels grow over the iris, preventing the eye fluid from draining normally. It is referred to as a "secondary" glaucoma because an underlying disease causes it.

Glucose: Blood sugar.

Glycosylated hemoglobin: Also called hemoglobin A1c or HbA1c. *See also* Hemoglobin A1c.

H

Hard exudates: Cholesterol and other fatty deposits that originate from the fluid that leaked into the retina, causing small waxy yellow dots that can be seen during an eye exam.

Hemoglobin A1C: Also called HbA1c or glycosylated hemoglobin is a key blood test in determining how well your diabetes treatment is working. Hemoglobin is a substance within the red blood cells that carries oxygen throughout the body. In uncontrolled diabetes it becomes "glycosylated" or combined with built-up sugar. With a periodic hemoglobin A1c test, a doctor can measure the average levels of sugar in the blood. Higher levels over time mean greater complication risks.

HDL (high-density lipoproteins): The "good" form of cholesterol that removes cholesterol from the body.

High blood pressure: An elevation of the pressure of blood in the arteries produced by the pumping action of the heart.

Hyperglycemia: High blood sugar.

Hypertension: A condition also known as high blood pressure.

Hypoglycemia: Blood sugar level that is lower than normal levels. Hypoglycemia may cause light-headedness and loss of consciousness.

I

Infection: Inflammation in body tissue caused by microorganisms.

Inflammation: A natural response in the body to fight disease and infections that, when it becomes chronic, is associated with increased risk for disease.

Insulin: Hormone produced by the pancreas necessary to convert sugar (*glucose*) into energy in the body. In type 1 diabetes the body does not produce it; in type 2 diabetes the body does not respond well to the insulin produced by the pancreas.

Internal limiting membrane: Thin layer covering the inner surface of the retina. It represents the boundary between the retina and the vitreous gel.

Intraocular lens: Type of artificial lens implanted during cataract surgery.

Intraocular pressure: Pressure within the eye.

Intravitreal injection: Injection into the vitreous, or middle, of the eye. Intravitreal injections of various drugs are frequently used forms of treatment for diabetic retinopathy and macular degeneration.

Iris: The tissue in front of the lens that opens and closes to control the amount of light entering the eye. The iris is the structure that gives color to the eye.

K

Kidney: The organ that helps filter waste from the blood stream and produce urine. Patients with kidney failure often need dialysis.

L

Laser photocoagulation: A treatment for diabetic retinopathy that involves the use of a laser light. Focal laser photocoagulation is used to treat diabetic macular edema. Panretinal laser photocoagulation is applied in a scatter pattern when new vessel growth has caused damage to the peripheral retina in proliferative diabetic retinopathy.

Lens: The clear structure near the front of the eye that focuses images onto the retina. It has the same function as the lens within a camera.

LDL (low-density lipoproteins): The "bad" form of cholesterol that is more likely to form the plaques that can block arteries.

Lipids: Fats in the body, including cholesterol.

Lipoproteins: Molecules of protein and fat that carry cholesterol through the bloodstream.

Low vision: Term used to denote reduced vision that cannot be corrected with glasses or contact lenses.

Lutein: A micronutrient that protects retinal cells from damage.

M

Macula: The center of the retina. The macula is responsible for direct and detailed focusing, and perception of colors.

Macular degeneration: Macular degeneration involves degenerative changes in the macula that may lead to loss of central vision. It is the most common cause of legal blindness among people over age fifty. *See also* Age-related macular degeneration.

Macular edema: Swelling of the macula caused by an accumulation of fluid from leaky blood vessels.

Macular ischemia: Lack of sufficient blood flow to the macula caused by the closure of small vessels in the retina. Vision blurs because the macula no longer receives enough nourishment to work properly.

Macular pucker: A thin membrane growing on the retina that contracts and distorts the retina, resulting in blurred and distorted vision. *See also* Epiretinal membrane.

Microaneurysms: Small bulges in the retinal blood vessels that leak fluid. These protrusions are the early signs of diabetic retinopathy.

Microscope: An instrument that provides magnified images of very tiny objects.

Monounsaturated fat: A group of fats that are better for the body than saturated or polyunsaturated fats. Olive oil and canola oil are good sources of monounsaturated fats.

N

Neovascular glaucoma: Pressure build-up inside the eye caused by abnormal new vessel growth over the iris.

Neovascularization: The formation of new abnormal blood vessels. Diabetes is the leading cause of retinal neovascularization, and wet macular degeneration is the leading cause of choroidal neovascularization.

Nerves: Cells that convey impulses to and from the central nervous system and other parts of the body.

O

Ophthalmologist: A physician (medical doctor) who specializes in the diagnosis, medical treatment, and surgical treatment of eye diseases.

Ophthalmoscope: A device used to visualize the retina.

Ophthalmoscopy: Examination of the structures at the back of the eye using an ophthalmoscope.

Optical character recognition: Software program that converts text from books, magazines, newspapers, and other paper articles into a form that a computer can read and edit.

Optical coherence tomography (OCT): A diagnostic test that uses light technology to produce a high-resolution scan of the macula or other ocular structures.

Optic nerve: A nerve that transmits visual information from the eye to the brain.

Optometrist: A licensed eye care professional who specializes in eye exams, prescribing lenses, and certain medical diagnoses and treatments.

P

Peripheral retina: The side areas of the retina.

Peripheral vision: Side vision.

Phacoemulsification: The surgical technique for removing a cataract by breaking or liquefying the affected lens with a special probe and then removing pieces via suction.

Photoreceptors: Retinal cells that detect light and send the information to the brain, where images and colors are perceived.

Polyunsaturated fats: A group of fats that help rid the body of cholesterol, but should still be limited in one's diet.

Pupil: Black circular part of the eye in the center of the iris that changes in size to regulate the amount of light entering the eye.

R

Retina: The part of the eye that contains the rods and the cones, specialized photoreceptor cells that receive an image from the lens and convey visual information to the brain via the optic nerve. The retina functions much like the film in a camera.

Retinal detachment: A separation of the retina from the back of the eye that requires medical attention. "Tractional retinal detachment," which can occur in diabetic retinopathy, involves abnormal tissue and blood vessels growing between the surface of the retina and back part of the vitreous and pulling the retina away.

Retinal hemorrhage: Tiny blood spots due to leakage of blood into the retina.

Retinal pigment epithelium (RPE): A single layer of cells between the retina and the underlying choroid.

Retina specialist: An ophthalmologist specializing in diseases of the retina.

Risk factors: Factors that increase a person's risk of getting a disease.

S

Saturated fats: Fats found in red meats and certain plants, such as coconut and palm. High levels of these fats are known to be harmful to the body and should be limited.

Slit lamp: A modified microscope with a bright light used for examining the eye.

Snellen eye chart: Chart that typically contains rows of gradu-ated-sized letters; it is used to test visual acuity.

Symptom: What you experience because of a disease such as poor vision.

T

Tear film: A layer of fluid that bathes and lubricates the cornea.

Tonometry: Test that measures intraocular pressure or pressure inside the eye.

Trabecular meshwork: Network of tiny canals through which eye fluid drains.

Trans fat (trans fatty acids): The unhealthy result of artificial process of "hydrogenating" or converting vegetable oil into a more stable form. Trans fatty acids are known to increase "bad" cholesterol, reduce "good" cholesterol, and overall contribute to the increase in heart-causing arterial plaque.

Triglycerides: Fat found in animal and plant fats and oils. Considered a risk factor for heart disease if consumed in excess. The fasting blood test that measures cholesterol usually measures triglyceride levels also.

20/20 vision: Normal visual acuity. First number indicates the standard distance (twenty feet) from the eye chart. Second number indicates the ability to identify the line on the chart that a normally sighted individual can identify from twenty feet away.

U

Ultraviolet (UV) light: The nonvisible portion of the light spectrum with a wavelength shorter than violet light.

V

Vascular endothelial growth factor (VEGF): A type of protein that stimulates the growth of abnormal blood vessels.

Visual acuity: A measure of the clarity of one's vision.

Visual field: A test used to measure areas of vision.

Vitrectomy: Surgical removal of the vitreous gel.

Vitreous: The clear, jelly-like substance in the central portion of the eye.

Vitreous hemorrhage: Hemorrhage within the vitreous of the eye.

W

Wet macular degeneration: A type of macular degeneration characterized by choroidal neovascularization causing leakage of fluid and bleeding under the retina and loss of central vision.

Z

Zeaxanthin: A nutrient that may protect against macular degeneration, but which has not yet been proven to do so.

Zinc: An antioxidant that neutralizes free radicals and is important to the proper functioning of the body.

Index

About the Authors

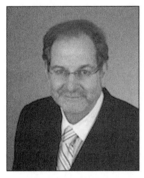 **David S. Boyer, M.D.,** is a world-renowned clinician, surgeon, and educator. He is the medical director of Retina-Vitreous Associates Medical Group in southern California. Dr. Boyer currently is a leading investigator for various national clinical trials on retinal diseases and serves as an advisor for numerous research, educational, and charitable institutions.

Dr. Boyer received his bachelor of science degree from the University of Illinois at Champaign, after which he completed his medical degree at the Chicago Medical School. In 1976, he finished his residency at the USC County Medical Center in Los Angeles. He completed his training with a retina fellowship at Wills Eye Hospital in Philadelphia.

Dr. Boyer has been a contributing author to many pivotal publications describing new treatments for retinal diseases.

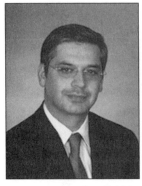

Homayoun Tabandeh, M.D., M.S., F.R.C.P., F.R.C.Ophth., is an internationally recognized retina specialist, in practice with Retina-Vitreous Associates Medical Group. He has authored more than 150 journal articles, book chapters, and abstracts and has extensive experience in the field of retinal disorders.

Dr. Tabandeh trained at three world-renowned eye institutes. He completed his residency in ophthalmology at the Wilmer Eye Institute, Johns Hopkins Hospital, in Baltimore and spent three years in retina fellowships at the Bascom Palmer Eye Institute in Miami and Moorfields Eye Hospital in London.

Dr. Tabandeh has been an investigator in many national and international clinical trials for the treatment of retinal diseases and has received awards in research, education, and patient care. Dr. Tabandeh previously served as the director of the Retina Service, Department of Ophthalmology, University of Florida, in Gainesville.

Consumer Health Titles from Addicus Books

Visit our online catalog at www.AddicusBooks.com

To Order Books:
Visit us online at: www.AddicusBooks.com
Call toll free: (800) 352-2873

For discounts on bulk purchases, call our Special Sales
Department at (402) 330-7493.
Or email us at: info@Addicus Books.com

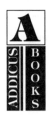

Addicus Books
P. O. Box 45327
Omaha, NE 68145

*Addicus Books is dedicated to publishing consumer health books
that comfort and educate.*